What Should I Eat?

Book 2 - Food as Medicine

Rudy Scarfalloto DC, DCBCN, DCCN

ISBN-13: 978-1717387639

ISBN-10: 1717387632

LCCN: 2018905081



Serenity Press

Cover image by Charles Cimarik

**Disclaimer**

The information is this book is for educational purposes only and is not
intended as a substitute for medical treatment. Individuals experiencing
health problems are advised to seek the advice and services of a medical
doctor or other qualitied health professionals.

# Other Books by Rudy Scarfalloto

*The Dance of Opposites*

*Cultivating Inner Harmony*

*The Edge of Time*

*Nutrition for Massage Therapists*

*What Should I Eat? Book 1— Finding Your Ideal Diet*

# Acknowledgments

My thanks to Jeremy Taylor, Deborah Dewberry and Sasha Snyder and Judith Steinman for their editorial assistance. My thanks to Linda Westman, Susan Pepka, and Sarah Anne Kaberah for their helpful suggestions. My thanks to Donna Overall, Mark Gandomkar, Michael Zollinger and Sunny Aasgaard for their contribution to the cover design. My thanks to Laura Fratto for the illustration on page 61. My Thanks to Chuck Cimarik for photographing the heart image on the cover. Special thanks to Leslie Marcinek and Chuck Cimarik — my heart-creation crew — for their enthusiastic participation in crafting the real-life fruit-and-vegetable masterpiece which has become the cover image of this book.

# Readers' Comments

"Dr. Scarfalloto is a brilliant leader in the field of nutrition. This book will become your most trusted nutritional reference. It is excellent, thorough, cutting-edge and has an unusually valuable bibliography." ~ Doris Helge, Ph.D. Author of *Transforming Pain into Power* and other works.

"Once again, Dr. Scarfalloto has taken complex ideas and conflicted beliefs about food and transformed them into easily understood and useful concepts. This book beautifully illustrates how one's food choices can either enhance or degrade one's health, and not necessarily as we were taught to believe. I say this because I have been in the health field for over forty years, during which I have been studying and writing about nutrition — and this book has still been an eye opener, compelling me to take a fresh look at some established ideas about food and nutrition." ~ Howard L. Silverman, Ph.D., D.C., D.A.B.C.T.

*"What Should I Eat? Book 2 — Food as Medicine* takes a unique and refreshing look at food and health. Here, readers will find nothing preachy or stale. It is ideal for health-seeking individuals and clinicians alike. A huge part of its appeal is that it avoids the pit-falls of 'one size fits all' thinking. Dr. Scarfalloto is mindful of physiological diversity and personal nutritional needs. The appendices alone are worth the price of this book. This is the sort of book you can return to again and again to find answers to your nutritional questions." ~Vista K. McCroskey, Ph.D., CHHC

"I really enjoyed this book. The author's writing style is easy to follow, his explanations are clear, and his sense of humor, delightful. Thank you, Dr Scarfalloto." ~ Marilyn Bradley LMT

*"What Should I Eat Book 2* is a must for those who want to use food to prevent or reverse illness. I would especially recommend it for the person caregiving for an ADD, ADHD, or a neurologically ill individual." ~ Sara Ann Butler, CCC/SLP voice coach.

"This book is so good! Unlike many nutritional books on the market, this one clearly presents the science behind the various food choices. Using Dr. Scarfalloto's suggestions, I have lost weight at a rate that is perfect for me. I expect this book will continue to serve me well as I pursue the long distance running that I love." ~ Sasha Snyder, MA, MLIS

I love this book! I feel it can provide new hope for individuals with health challenges, as it did for me. One of my favorite features is the inclusion of framed "sound-bites" which encapsulate the central idea of the preceding section. I am using this organizational aid to guide me in my use of food. Another feature I appreciate is that you can use this book on several levels: you can use it as a reference book to quickly look up information or read it more thoroughly for deeper understanding. In addition to providing practical information on nutrition and health, I feel that this book can touch the reader on emotional and spiritual levels. This is the sort of book that you can read over and over again, and each time it will bring new insights. ~ Rev. Judith Steinman

"Expanding on *What Should I Eat? Book 1,* this book shows us how food and diets can cause, prevent, or reverse specific illnesses. As in *Book 1,* the author is not one sided. He helps us discover which foods and diets would work best for our personal health needs. This is a great book for someone starting their journey to good health or for someone looking to bring together the jumble of diet ideas that are out there." ~ Jeremy Taylor, BA, LMT, NMT

'This book may save your life. It offers a real-world antidote to the public health crisis caused by mass-consumption of processed and denatured food. The chapter on cancer alone is worth the price of the book. Thoughtful and brilliantly researched, this book is an absorbing read, combining clear and concise physiology, up-to-date nutritional science, and what seems to me to be an intuitive understanding of food, health, and disease. With all its strong points, its most striking gift is the simplicity it advocates: a pharmacopeia at everyone's disposal — whole, unprocessed foods at the local farmer's market." ~ Deborah Dewberry, M.A., journalist, and promotor of Wellness Programs for the ACCG Health Benefits Plan.

# How to Use this Book

There are three basic ways in which you may use this book.

- **Quick reference.** You may use the General Index at the end of the book to quickly look up any subject of interest. You may also use the Food as Medicine Index which directs you to the page or pages describing specific nutritional support for a given health challenge.

- **Deeper learning**. You may read a specific chapter which gives the details on health issues that are of interest to you. Each chapter is self-contained; therefore, you may go directly to the one that addresses a given topic, without necessarily reading the preceding chapters. In addition, the appendix provides a guide for food-related topics that are controversial, confusing or of special interest.

- **Deepest learning**. If you first read chapters 1-5 in the order presented, you will receive the foundational knowledge which will allow you to get the most out of the remainder of the book.

# Contents

# Introduction

*"Let food be your medicine and medicine your food."*
*— Hippocrates*

Most health care practitioners would agree with Hippocrates' admonishment to use food as medicine, at least in theory. However, to put Hippocrates' principle into practice is not as easy as it might seem; and is probably more challenging today than it was in ancient Greece. That is why I have written the present book.

As you might guess from the title, this book could be described as the sequel to *What Should I Eat, Book 1* which is about healthy eating in general. *Book 2* uses the same core principles described in *Book 1* and applies them to help prevent and possibly reverse the health issues associated with modern living. However, you need not read *Book 1* in order to apply *Book 2*, because the latter provides a review of the fundamentals in *Book 1*.

## The Doctor as Teacher

Hippocrates' principle about the use of food to restore health implies that he did not merely treat his patients and then send them home with a bag of herbs or potions. His view of the role of the physician included *teaching* patients how to restore and maintain health. This might be why practitioners who followed in Hippocrates footsteps came to be known as "doctors." The original meaning of this word translates into "teacher."

Over the centuries, the role of physicians as teachers of health has become increasingly marginalized. The typical "successful" doctor of today seems too busy to talk with his patients about restoring and maintaining health.

Fortunately, the general public is awakening to the realization that health does not come from the medicine cabinet, nor from the physician who is too busy to teach patients how to restore and maintain health.

More and more health-conscious individuals are seeking health care providers who understand that the word "doctor" means teacher. Such awareness is creating a demand for physicians who would follow in the footsteps of Hippocrates.

Granted, there is a legitimate place for the methods used by conventional Western medicine today. Western medicine is superb at saving a person's life during a crisis. However, many of these crises are preventable. Even when someone does get seriously ill, recovery can often be greatly facilitated by having the person make nutritional and lifestyle adjustments. Many of these nutritional measures are quite simple and are described throughout this book.

# Chapter 1
# Food for Thought

The Two Sides of Clear Thinking
Obstacles to Clear Thinking
In Summary


*"It ain't what you don't know that gets you into trouble.*
*It's what you know for sure that just ain't so."*
*— Mark Twain*


Lack of objectivity is a stumbling block in the study of nutrition, resulting in much arguing among its teachers and confusion among the health-seeking public. To complicate matters, objectivity can be especially challenging in the study of diets and nutrition because food tends to be a rather emotional subject. Hence this chapter.

When objectivity is lacking, we appear to ask questions but secretly assume that we already know the answer. We seem to seek the truth but might really be defending our beliefs.

The good news is that objectivity does not require us to be totally free of emotional leaning. Neither do we have to be intellectually gifted or obtain a university degree. You don't have to be a scientist to think like one. As Albert Einstein point out, science is just the refinement of everyday thinking.

Such refinement of thinking is available to everyone. The only requirement is that our primary loyalty is to the truth. In other words, the capacity to be objective arises naturally with the willingness to be honest with oneself. Yes, it is that simple.

However, *simple* is not the same as *easy*. As civilized humans, we are exposed to a number of stressors that tempt and seduce us to abandon objectivity and evert our eyes from the truth. This chapter provides some simple ways to polish the lens of our intellect and cultivate clear thinking and objectivity, so that we can make sense of the nutritional information we encounter.

> The foundation for clear thinking is the willingness to be
> honest with oneself.

# The Two Sides of Clear Thinking

If we wish to think more clearly and objectively, we can do so by first recognizing that objectivity has two sides: caution and candor. Caution means that we refrain from jumping to conclusions. Candor means that we bring to light all relevant information, rather than censoring data that might go against our pre-existing beliefs.

Caution and candor are synergistic. Together, they are the Yin and Yang of clear thinking. Caution compels us to be still and hold our peace. Candor compels us to proactively bring forth all relevant data. This is how we cultivate intellectual honesty, wherein we patiently refrain from drawing hasty conclusions, taking time to consider all pertinent information.

Caution and candor are the foundation of good science. Together, they keep us mentally alert, as well as providing a reality-check if we happen to drift into mental laziness or wishful thinking. Together, they sharpen our power of discernment, allowing us to distinguish solid nutritional data from a slick sales pitch wearing a white lab coat.

| Caution and candor are the foundation of good science. |
| --- |

# Obstacles to Clear Thinking

Beyond exercising caution and candor, we may further deepen our capacity for clear thinking by recognizing some of the common ways in which we drift away from it, as described below.

## Reductionist Thinking Gone Bad

Western science is good at dissecting things to identify the individual pieces of whatever we are studying. This is called reductionism.

Reductionist thinking is useful — as long as we recognize its limitations! One limitation is that the very act of breaking things down to their fundamental components can easily cause us to lose sight of the whole. When we focus to closely on the fragments, our thinking becomes fragmented. We fixate on the pieces and fail to appreciate the importance of relationship. We fail to see the interdependence of the parts. This can be particularly problematical in the study of nutrition, because good nutrition is all about relationship.

Understanding the subtleties of good nutrition is about recognizing the countless nutrients which dance harmoniously within the physiological milieu of the body. In order for them to do so, they must be present in the right proportions. For example, there is a huge difference in the way the body handles carbohydrates in white bread or refined sugar compared to carbohydrates in whole foods which are synergistically combined with vitamins, minerals, phytonutrients, and fiber.

Lack of appreciation for the bigger picture is one of the occupational hazards of Western science in general. In the study of nutrition, we might unconsciously assume that a given nutrient behaves the same in the body as it does in a test tube. We assume a give nutrient is handled by the body in the same, whether it is ingested in isolation or as part of a whole food matrix. Apparently there is a huge difference! For example, beta carotene has been shown to have a number of benefits, including protection from cancer. However, when removed from its whole food matrix, and given in high doses, it has been found to *increase* the risk of lung cancer in smokers.[1] Similarly, vitamin C offers antioxidant protection when consumed in whole foods but can *increase* oxidative stress when consumed as an isolated nutrient![2]

> Good nutrition is about relationship.

## Jumping to Conclusions

Losing sight of the relationship factor is just one of the ways that we trick ourselves into jumping to conclusions. When we jump to conclusions, good science becomes bad science. When we jump to conclusions, we forget that reality is not necessarily the same as our perception of it. We forget that the horizon is not the end of the world, but simply marks the limit of our sight. We assume that the nutritional information that we happen to possess is all the information which is relevant.

Jumping to conclusions often translates into short-sightedness, wherein we think only in terms of immediate results, and do not consider the long-term consequences of our actions. This is a huge stumbling block in nutrition. It is also a stumbling block in healthcare in general. Many health seekers and health professionals fall into this trap. For example, we might take a drug to resolve one problem, but do not consider the long-term consequences for the rest of the body. In the diet world, many individuals go on a high-protein diet to rapidly lose weight, without considering the long-term consequences of such a diet — which can be harmful, as described in the next chapter. This is where the old cliché, "a little knowledge is dangerous," is all too true.

Beyond the desire to lose weight quickly, many individuals overestimate the dietary need for protein. This assumption dates back to the late 19th century, when researchers discovered that the dry weight of the body is mostly protein. Therefore, they *assumed* that a healthy diet should be rich in protein.

The assumption that humans need lots of protein quickly found its way to the general public, where it eventually became so deeply entrenched that it persists to the present day. This assumption has persisted even after subsequent research repeatedly showed that our protein requirements are rather modest; and that any surplus contributes to rapid aging and degeneration, as described in the next chapter.

Another assumption among some students of nutrition is the notion that sugar in fresh fruit contributes to tumor growth and therefore fruit should be avoided by individuals undergoing cancer treatment. This idea is based on the fact that sugar does indeed feed cancer cells. However, the assumption about fresh fruit promoting tumor growth ignores several other facts. For example, our blood sugar (glucose) doesn't just feed cancer cells, it feeds *all* our body cells. In addition, the assumption about fruit and tumor growth ignores the fact that fresh fruit contains a wealth of other nutrients which have been shown to help the body prevent or reverse tumor growth, as described in chapter 14.

Another common way in which we jump to conclusions in the study of nutrition is the unspoken assumption that a good short-term therapeutic diet for a given individual is also a good maintenance diet for *everyone.* This assumption is pervasive in the diet world it because usually goes unrecognized and is therefore unchallenged. In other words, a certain diet might show promise in resolving a specific health challenge in some individuals − and on that basis, it is promoted as an appropriate long-term diet for everyone! This is a common way that many diets are promoted to the public.

> One source of confusion about healthy eating is the unspoken assumption that a good therapeutic diet for some individuals is also a good maintenance diet for *everyone.*

Jumping to conclusions has also occurred in agriculture, with devastating results on the quality of food. In his book, *The Omnivore's Dilemma,* Michael Pollan describes how farmers in the early 20th century were encouraged to abandon traditional methods of growing food in favor of chemical fertilizers, pesticides, and eventually herbicides. This was based on grossly simplistic assumptions about soil, as Pollan explains:

> "...To reduce such a vast biological complexity (soil) to NPK (nitrogen, phosphorus and potassium fertilizers) represents the scientific method at its reductionist worst. Complex qualities are reduced to simple quantities; biology gives way to chemistry...The problem is that once science has reduced a complex phenomenon to a couple of variables, the tendency is to overlook everything else, to assume that what you measure is all that there is, or at least all that really matters. When we mistake what we can know for all there is to know, a healthy appreciation for one's ignorance in the face of a mystery, like soil fertility, gives way to the hubris that we can treat nature as a machine."[3]

Pollan goes on to explain how chemical fertilizers make plants more vulnerable to marauding insects and disease, so that farmers must turn to chemical pesticides to fix the problem. They eventually noted that their pastures and animals had become less robust. In retrospect, we can understand why this occurred: chemical fertilizers deplete minerals from the soil, resulting in reduction of the health promoting properties of food. Food grown on synthetically fertilized soil is less nourishing than food grown in composted soil.[4] This is not the sort of food we would favor if we were seriously interested in using food to help recover from illness.

> "When we mistake what we can know for all there is to know, a healthy appreciation for one's ignorance...gives way to the hubris that we can treat nature as a machine."

Pollan reminds us that good science must include what he calls "a health appreciation for the unknown." This is also good advice for anyone who wants to understand nutrition or who just wants to able think clearly. Such wisdom was also voiced thousands of years ago by the Chinese philosopher Confucius who said, "The greatest knowledge is knowledge of ones own ignorance."

## Treating Science as Religion
Science is at its best when we make a clear distinction between facts and theories. The moment that a theory is promoted to the

status of an unquestioned belief, science is no longer science; it is operating in the realm of religion. For example, in 1952, James Watson and Francis Crick published their groundbreaking research that suggested DNA is the carrier of genetic information. However, they interpreted the data in such a way which assumes the information in DNA to be fixed — that it cannot be influenced by environmental factors, such as food.[5] Their theory was so persuasive, that Dr. Crick eventually proclaimed that their model of inheritance was "the central dogma" of biology.

"Dogma" implies the idea is beyond question. And indeed, for many years, the central dogma of biology was unchallenged, and any biologist who seriously questioned it was risking his or her credibility and would essentially be "excommunicated."

One of the consequences regarding the perceived supremacy of DNA was to underestimate the value of food and disempowered the individual. The theory basically says that we are puppets on a string — in this case, strands of DNA. In reality, food can be powerful medicine, even with conditions that are technically genetic in origin. Food can have a profound effect on gene expression, wherein a "genetic weakness" does not have to manifest as an actual disease.

> Food can be powerful medicine, even with conditions that are technically genetic in origin.

## Misusing the Absence of Evidence

Good science responds to lack of evidence by simply withholding judgment. However, science-minded individuals often reject an idea because of lack of hard evidence. This is the antithesis of good science but it is commonly used to give an argument a scientific veneer. For example, in the latter part of the 20th century, when a growing number of dentists, researchers, and health consumers voiced concern about the use of mercury in dental fillings, critics often tried to dismiss these concerns by saying something like, "There is no scientific evidence to support the theory that mercury amalgam fillings are harmful."

Even if there is no hard evidence to support a given theory, a good scientist might still give it thoughtful consideration if there is enough anecdotal evidence in favor of it, such as clinical reports and testimonials. For example, the theory of food combining – the idea that combining foods in a given manner can benefit digestion –

has been rejected or ridiculed by some critics because no double-blind, placebo-controlled, randomized studies exist which support it. However, there is no shortage of anecdotal evidence on the subject, including positive clinical results.

## Comparing Our Strengths with Their Weaknesses

Focusing on the weakest part of an argument is a common tactic in debates. This is known as the "straw-man" argument. The attack on the opposition's weakness is often followed by highlighting one's own strong points. In other words, we shine a light on their weaknesses and our strengths — their failures and our successes — while ignoring the other side of the coin.

We often do this unconsciously and with the best of intentions, and therefore feel justified in adopting highly polarized beliefs, wherein we passionately see no goodness in the other party's teachings, and no fault in our own. For example, promoters of low-carb diets often begin their presentation by pointing to problems with over-consuming carbohydrates. This is often followed by success stories of individuals on a low-carb diet. Meanwhile, the competition is using the exact same strategy!

This is why we can listen to one diet promoter who seems very persuasive, and then listen to another who says the opposite — but sounds equally persuasive! Very confusing indeed, until we see the fallacy in this sort of argument.

> Shining a light on ones strengths and their weaknesses, while ignoring the other side of the coin, is common in diet debates.

## False Dichotomies

A false dichotomy refers to artificially created opposing viewpoints wherein we impose either/or restrictions on an issue that isn't necessarily either/or. For example, "You are either with us or against us." We see this a lot in the world of politics where the public is given just two (mutually exclusive) choices to address a given issue, to the exclusion of all others. Such an argument denies the possibility of neutrality. It also ignores other options besides the two being presented.

False dichotomies are common in the diet world. For example, the question regarding the proper place of animal products in human nutrition has often been polarized into strict vegan vs. a meat-rich omnivorous diet. Furthermore, each option is often presented in a way which assumes that *all* humans should eat that way. In other words, this dichotomy assumes that good nutrition is one-size-fits-all. It also overlooks the possibility of eating mostly plant foods with relatively modest amounts of animal products, adjusted to the needs of the individual. For example, some individuals might eat vegan on most days, punctuated by the occasional use of animal products.

> A false dichotomy ignores other options besides the two being presented.

## Emotional Attachment

We can become emotionally attached to a dietary theory, just as we can become attached to some foods. Such attachment can obviously undermine our intention to be objective. It can make us intolerant of other viewpoints and preferences. Such attachment also makes it difficult to change one's mind in the presence of new evidence. In fact, it can cause us to (perhaps unconsciously) avoid looking at any data which might challenge our beliefs.

The good news is that we need not struggle with our preferences. The simple awareness of our emotional leanings might be all we need to make rational decisions. For example, for the past 16 years or so, I have been eating a fruit-based diet, which means that the bulk of my calories come from fruit. In my early years of eating this way, I noticed that if I happened to encounter information that criticized this sort of diet, or claimed to "debunk" it, I was tempted to discard the information, because I found it too unsettling. Fortunately, as is often the case in such situations, my defensiveness started dissolving when I simply recognized it. It dissolved even more when I reminded myself that it's okay if I don't have all the answers at the present moment and it's okay if I discover that I need to change my diet in the future. Yes, we are talking about freedom here.

> It's okay to change your mind in the presence of new evidence.

## The Need to Belong

The emotional need for belonging is another subtle factor that can dissuade us from thinking outside the box. The need to belong makes us conform. It makes us turn away from ideas that are not acceptable in our social circle. The need to belong is powerful, perhaps reflecting an ancestral memory of a time when personal survival depended on belonging to a tribe. In some tribal societies, such as those described in the Bible, banishment was considered equal to or worse than death.

The emotional need to belong has a presence in the diet world. A major change in diet might threaten personal identity and close relationships. Such "imprinting" can happen insidiously every time we read a book or attend a party. It can occur on an even deeper level at long conference or symposium, where useful information becomes a vehicle for indoctrination and emotional bonding with other members — similar to a religious revival or political convention.

## In Summary

All the impediments to clear thinking described in this chapter tend to fall away by just recognizing them. This is how the mind can become free and open, so we are willing to bring forth all pertinent information (candor), rather than conveniently ignoring data that don't support our beliefs. With equal ease, we become more inclined to hold our peace and refrain from jumping to conclusions (caution), when faced with new data.

Objectivity means that our primary loyalty is to the truth, not to any particular dietary doctrine. Objectivity means that the mind remains alert, flexible and curious. We do not put on blinders. We do not cherry-pick data and give its "spin" so as to validate our preexisting beliefs. Neither do we drift into a jaded complacency wherein we assume to know all there is to know about a given subject.

When we practice objectivity, our thinking becomes clear and precise so that it resembles that of a scientist. The mind of a true scientist has the unrestricted curiosity of a child. Such a mind is free to think outside the box. In a subtle kind of way, when we practice objectivity, we enliven and rejuvenate the mind.

---

To be objective means that your primary loyalty is to the truth.

---

# Chapter 2
# Food as Food

What *is* a Balanced Diet?
How Does Food Make Us Sick?
What is Whole Food?
Variety and Simplicity
The Food Groups
*Your* Ideal Diet

The first step in using food as medicine is to understand how it differs from using food as food. Using food as food may be likened to owning a small boat; all you have to do is clean it, paint or varnish it once in a while, and refrain from doing anything that might interfere with its buoyancy. On the other hand, using food as medicine may be likened to having a boat that has a hole in it; now you have to bail out the water and patch up the hole in a timely manner before the boat is swallowed by the sea.

In other words, using food as food means our goal is to *maintain* health, while using food as medicine means our goal is to *restore* health. The two are related, of course. To safely and effectively use food as medicine, you must first establish a solid foundation — the proper use of food for everyday nourishment.

Using food to maintain health is as simple as eating a balanced diet. Yes, it is that simple — if we have a clear idea of what constitutes a balanced diet. The use of food for everyday nourishment is the subject of my other book, *What Should I Eat? Book 1 – Finding Your Ideal Diet.* The essential elements of that book are summarized below.

## What *is* a Balanced Diet?

Health-conscious individuals frequently use the term, balanced diet, but often in vague or nebulous ways. What exactly are we endeavoring to "balance?" The short answer is that we are endeavoring to balance our intake of nutrients. Therefore, to understand what constitutes a balanced diet, we need to first gain a basic understanding of the six major classes of nutrients.

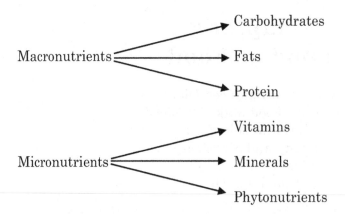

Carbohydrates, fats and protein are called *macronutrients* because we consume them in relatively large amounts. In contrast, vitamins, minerals, and phytonutrients are called *micronutrients* because they are consumed in relatively small amounts. Typically, the food on your plate is dominated by carbohydrates, fats, and protein, while the vitamins, minerals and phytonutrients can fit on a teaspoon.

Some nutrients are needed in greater amounts than others because of their different roles in the body. The roles played by nutrients are vast and complex, but there is an underlying simplicity: any molecule that serves as a nutrient will be used by the body in at least one of three ways:

- It is burned as fuel.
- It is used as building material.
- It helps to regulate the body.

When a nutrient is burned as fuel, it is broken down to release energy, which is measured in *calories*. In contrast, when a nutrient is used as building material, its molecules are not broken down, but joined together like bricks to form muscles, bones, internal organs, skin, etc. When nutrients are used for regulation, they are neither burned nor assembled, but rather used to help direct the workings of the body.

Once we recognize the three basic ways that the body uses nutrients, we can also understand why some of them are "macro," while others are "micro." Carbohydrates, fats, and protein are needed in relatively large amounts because they are used primarily as fuel or as building material. In that capacity, they are used up rather quickly and must be replenished in a timely manner.

In contrast, vitamins, minerals, and phytonutrients are needed in much smaller amounts because they are typically not burned for energy or assembled as building material. Instead, they are used primarily for regulation, which usually means that the same molecules can be used over and over again.

## A closer look at macronutrients

- **Carbohydrates** are used primarily as fuel. The two main forms of carbohydrates are sugars and complex carbohydrates.
- **Protein** is used primarily as building material to make the flesh of the body, as well as to make enzymes and hormones.
- **Fats** are burned for energy and used as building material. Some fats are also used to make hormones.

## A closer look at micronutrients

Since micronutrients are used mostly for regulation, they are the key to maintaining and restoring health. In that regard, the quality of the food we eat makes a big difference. For example, vitamins and minerals are often removed when foods are processed, as with refined sugar, white rice, and white bread. Likewise, there is a big difference between farm-fresh meat, eggs and dairy derived from pasture-raised animals, compared to the same products derived from factory-raised animals raised on devitalized animal feed, laced with hormones and antibiotics.

| Micronutrients are the key to maintaining and restoring health. |
| --- |

Even without processing, foods that are picked one or two weeks prior to eating, especially vegetables, are likely to be depleted of many vitamins. and phytonutrients. This is why it is good to get as much food as possible from local growers.

Minerals are not perishable like vitamins and phytonutrients, but they do present another challenge. They are not made by the plant, like vitamins, but must be pulled out of the soil. As mentioned in the previous chapter, the use of artificial fertilizers depletes minerals from the soil.

Though micronutrients are needed in relatively small amounts, their regulatory power is hugely important for restoring and maintaining health. Therefore, if we are serious about using food to prevent and reverse disease, we would do well to get as much of our food as possible from growers who take care of the soil, especially its mineral content.

When we fully appreciate the importance of micronutrients, the term, "balanced diet," is no longer vague or nebulous. We now have a clear idea of exactly what we are attempting to balance — we are balancing macronutrients with micronutrients.

> To use food as medicine, get as much of it as possible from local growers who take care of the soil, especially its mineral content.

## How Does Food Make Us Sick?

There is now general agreement in the field of nutrition that virtually all the health issues of modern civilization can be caused or aggravated by the overconsumption of macronutrients and under consumption of micronutrients and fiber. Even when food is clearly not the primary cause of a given health problem, the changes of recovery can be greatly increased when food intake is optimized. In other words, a major reason that humans get sick or don't realize their potential for optimum health is because of ingesting too many calories, and not enough of the other nutritional elements. Yes, it really is that simple.

> A major cause or contributor to illness is the ingestion of too many calories and not enough vitamins, minerals, phytonutrients, and fiber.

Once we grasp the principle described above, we can see that a well-rounded diet offers the proper balance of macronutrients and micronutrients. The first and most important step to achieving such balance is to simply *favor whole foods*.

## What is Whole Food?

A food is considered "whole" when it contains all the nutrients that nature puts into it. For example, a banana is a whole food. On the other hand, cheese, tofu, vegetable oil and butter are not whole foods. They are extracts of whole foods.

I am not suggesting here that non-whole foods should be avoided. On the contrary, some of them may have good nutritive and even medicinal properties. However, moderation is advisable with non-whole foods because they tend to have high concentrations of some nutrients, while being deficient in others. Therefore, eating more than a modest amount of such foods can lead to nutritional imbalances.

One major issue with non-whole foods is that they tend to pack more calories than whole foods, resulting in unwanted weight gain. In addition, by consuming large amounts of calorically dense non-whole foods, we often marginalize other foods that we might need to round out our nutrition, resulting in multiple deficiencies.

Again, in making the distinction between whole foods and non-whole foods, my intention is not to vilify the latter, but to simply remind us to use non-whole foods conservatively, while favoring whole foods as the foundation of our meals.

> Healthy eating begins with whole foods as the foundation of our meals, while using non-whole foods more conservatively.

# Variety and Simplicity

Even with whole foods, variety is still important. By eating a wide variety of whole foods, the nutrients which are in short supply in one food can be provided by another.

Variety does not have to come with every meal. In fact, another useful concept for healthy eating, especially for good digestion, is to keep each meal fairly simple. Get your variety from meal to meal, day to day, and season to season.

The easiest way to get variety is to use all food groups, because each group has its own characteristic nutritional profile. This does not mean we absolutely *have* to include all food groups to have optimum health. It simply means that if we do choose to exclude one or more food groups, we should broaden our selection of the remaining groups. For example, if you exclude animal products, don't just eat more of the same grains and beans! Eat a wider variety of grains and beans, as well as including other plant foods, such as nuts and seeds, avocados, coconuts, mushrooms, and sea vegetation.

> For optimal digestion, keep each meal simple and get your variety from meal to meal, day to day, and season to season.

# The Food Groups

## Grains

- Grains include wheat, barley, rye, corn, rice, and oats.
- Grains tend to be high in calories, mostly in the form of starch.
- Most grains also have a substantial amount of protein. However, the protein found in some grains is called gluten, which can produce allergic reactions in some individuals.
- The tough outer covering of grains is made of a coarse fiber called bran, which is rich in vitamins and minerals. This is the main reason to favor whole grain products, such as whole wheat bread and brown rice, over refined grain products, such as white bread and white rice.

## Legumes

- Legumes include beans, peas, lentils, and peanuts.
- Legumes provide the bulk of their calories from carbohydrates, but also have substantial protein.
- Legumes tend to be rich in minerals, soluble fiber and various phytonutrients that promote stable blood sugar and protect against cardiovascular disease and cancer.
- The gas associated with legumes is from the presence of hard-to-digest carbohydrates. They can be reduced by soaking the legumes prior to cooking, as well as skimming off the starchy film on the surface of the water during cooking.

## Fruits

- A fruit is the fleshy covering around a seed.
- Most fruits are sweet because they are rich in sugars.
- Fruits tend to be rich in water, soluble fiber, vitamins, minerals, and phytonutrients.
- Fruits are cleansing to the body because of the ease of digestion, and high levels of fiber and water.
- Fruit is relatively low in calories, but still has enough to reduce our dependency on other foods, such as bread and meat, which require more digestive power and clean-up.

---

Fruit is a source of clean calories, thus reducing our dependency on other sources, such as wheat and meat, which require more digestion and clean-up.

---

## Vegetables

- The foods which we designate as vegetables typically consist of edible roots, stems, and leaves. In addition, some vegetables, such as cucumbers, tomatoes and bell peppers are actually botanical fruits but have a nutritional profile resembling that of leafy vegetables.
- A few vegetables, such as potatoes and winter squash, are rich in starch. The rest have a relatively low starch content. Therefore, they tend to be very low in calories, while still containing a wealth of vitamins, minerals, phytonutrients, and fiber.
- Because of their low caloric content and high levels of micronutrients and fiber, vegetables provide a powerful counterpoint to the high calorie foods that tend to dominate modern diets. This is why vegetables are Mother Nature's medicine.
- Because vegetables are the lowest in calories of all food groups. overeating vegetables is virtually impossible. For this reason, vegetables are valuable for individuals wanting to be moderate with their caloric intake, without becoming deficient in essential nutrients.

> Low-starch vegetables are Mother Nature's medicine because they are lowest in calories and highest in vitamins, minerals, phytonutrients, and fiber.

## Nuts and Seeds

- The foods we classify as nuts and seeds can generally be eaten raw, though roasting is a common practice. They include walnuts, almonds, sesame seeds and pumpkin seeds.
- Of all food groups, nuts, and seeds have the highest caloric content, mostly in the form of fat, with lesser amounts of carbohydrates and protein.

## Meat

- Meat comes from the muscles and internal organs of animals.
- Meat is high in calories, which come primarily from fat, secondarily from protein, with virtually no carbohydrates.
- Though meat provides the bulk of its calories from fat, the most striking contrast with plant foods is the much higher levels of protein in meat.

## Eggs

- Eggs are rich in, omega-3 oils, fat-soluble vitamins, saturated fats, and cholesterol.
- Factory-farmed eggs come from chickens raised under extremely unsanitary conditions. They are often loaded with antibiotics and are likely to be infected with salmonella.
- Eggs from free-range chickens are available in health food stores and some supermarkets. They are more nutritious than the factory farmed eggs. The best eggs have a rich, orange yolk.
- The consumption of eggs for maintaining and restoring health is currently a controversial topic. The details are given in Appendix A.

## Dairy

- Dairy includes milk, cheese, yogurt, kefir, and butter.
- Some individuals handle dairy fairly well. Many do not; they might have an allergy to the milk protein, or lack the enzyme needed to digest milk sugar.

# *Your* Ideal Diet

Author and food advocate Michael Pollan summarized healthy eating this way:

- Eat food
- Mostly plants
- Not too much[1]

Like Einstein's famous equation $e=mc^2$, Pollan's formula is brilliant in its simplicity. However, simple is not the same as easy. In this case, the very process of simplifying necessitates that we exclude a number of details. We can easily stumble over the details which are not mentioned, though implied, in Pollan's formula. These details have to do with *which* foods, *which* plants, and the specifics regarding *how* to not eat too much. The high incidence of obesity suggests that eating "not too much," though simple, is often far from easy. My other book, *What Should I Eat, Book 1*, fills in the details by providing the following principles:

**Your ideal diet is *your* ideal diet** and might be inappropriate for your friend or family member and vice versa.

**Your Ideal Diet can change with time** because your body changes with time.

**Your ideal diet is both rational and instinctual.** Rational means that your choices make sense to you and produce the desired results. Instinctual means that your choices feel right and the food tastes good. When intellect and instincts work together, the foods you love also love you back.

**Your ideal diet provides all nutrients in the cleanest and most digestible form available.** Digestion and clean-up use up a lot of energy and other resources. Therefore, by selecting the cleanest and most digestible foods, the energy which is conserved becomes available for other purposes, such as deeper cleansing and healing.

> Energy that isn't used to digest food can be used to digest diseases.

**Your ideal diet has a balance of building foods and cleansing foods.**[2] Building foods are high-calorie foods, such as grains, beans, nuts, seeds, and animal products. These foods are rich in protein, carbohydrates, and fats. Cleansing foods are fruits and leafy vegetables. Cleansing foods tend to be low in calories, and rich in vitamins, minerals, phytonutrients, fiber, and water.

Our food supply tends to encourage the overconsumption of building foods and under-consumption of cleansing foods, thus contributing to the onset of obesity and degenerative diseases, such as heart disease, cancer, and arthritis.

> Your ideal diet has a balance of building foods & cleansing foods.

**Your ideal diet balances acidifying and alkalizing foods.** Fruits and vegetables tend to alkalize the body. Animal products, grains, nuts, and seeds tend to be acid forming. This is not to suggest that alkalizing foods are good and acidifying foods are bad. Remember, acid-forming foods are also building foods – they contain high levels of nutritional elements needed to fuel and build the body. The key is balance. And the balance point can differ from one individual to another, which is why instincts and person experience are important in food selection.

**Your ideal diet is probably carb-based or fat-based.** Ideally, your instincts will guide you in this area without you having to give it much attention. However, if you have done all you can with regard to the above guidelines, but still have problems, the next step is to select your foods so you get most of your calories from carbohydrates, with fats relatively low, or vice versa. If you're not quite sure how to accomplish this, that's okay because virtually all the well-established dietary systems do this, though they usually do not call attention to it. Which one is best for you? The good news is that the right plan for you is the one that probably makes sense and feels right to you.

**Your ideal diet is part of a balanced life-style.** The instinctual side of eating is greatly influenced by our emotions. For most of us, food is a highly charged emotional issue. Food is a source of pleasure and comfort, as well as being an avenue through which we commune socially. This is normal and healthy. However, problems arise when we unconsciously attempt to use food to provide pleasure and comfort that we do not get from nurturing relationships and rewarding work. Granted, the right kind of food can help to promote mental clarity and emotional serenity, but it cannot cure loneliness.

Therefore, the choice to eat healthier implies that we also do what we can to invite fulfillment in other areas of life. By being responsive to our emotional needs, our food instincts are set free to do what they are designed to do — guide us in selecting health-giving foods.

### Bless Your Food

Blessing your food is a subtle but powerful way to change your relationship with it. It works even if you're agnostic! Blessing your food tends to relax the body and calm the mind. It is a way of remembering what is important in life. By getting into the habit of blessing your food and giving thanks before you eat it, you might be doing exactly what you need to do to properly apply Michael Pollan's three simple rules for healthy eating:

- Eat food
- Mostly plants
- Not too much

# Chapter 3
# Food as Medicine
## Part 1 – The Foods

The Physiology of Health
Healing Foods

This chapter is mostly a survey of foods which have been shown to have health-restoring properties. However, to fully appreciate how these foods can help maintain and restore health, we should first understand how the body normally maintains itself in a health state and recovers from illness. In other words, to understand how common foods can serve as medicine, let us look at the basic physiology and health and healing.

## The Physiology of Health

As you might guess, the details regarding how the body maintains and restores health can fill an entire book — and a very thick one at that! However, for the purpose of using food as medicine, we will presently focus on four features of restorative physiology:

- Inflammation
- Antioxidants
- Nitric oxide
- Glutathione

All four can be strongly influenced by food. In fact, the health promoting properties of the foods listed later in this chapter may be at least partially attributed to their effect on one or more of the four items listed above.

### Inflammation

Inflammation is the body's normal response to any irritant, whether in the form of physical injury, chemical toxicity, or infection. Inflammation includes increased blood flow, accumulation of fluids, and increased metabolism in the irritated tissue; all of which will help the body to cleanse and heal the affected area. This is why a sprained ankle becomes red and swollen.

On the downside, inflammation can also *cause* health problems if it lingers too long. Chronic low-grade inflammation is a common trigger for many diseases. In fact, most of the health problems described in this book have an inflammatory component.

Inflammation is greatly influenced by the kinds of foods we eat. This is one reason why virtually all degenerative diseases have a dietary connection to some degree.

Regarding inflammation and food, the bottom line is this: some foods are pro-inflammatory, while others are anti-inflammatory.[1] Studies suggest that we can prevent and sometimes reverse degenerative conditions, such as cardiovascular disease and arthritis, by adjusting the diet to include ample amounts of anti-inflammatory foods, while limiting pro-inflammatory foods.[2]

| Pro-inflammatory Foods | • Foods high in omega-6 oils, such as corn oil and soybean oil.<br>• Most grains and grain-fed beef.<br>• Dairy |
|---|---|
| Anti-inflammatory Foods | • Fruits<br>• Vegetables<br>• Foods rich in omega-3 oils: cold-water fish, flax seeds, chia seeds.<br>• Ginger, garlic, and turmeric |

## Antioxidants

Antioxidants neutralize free radicals. Free radicals are molecules that provoke the oxidation of other molecules. Oxidation is a chemical process by which some molecules are broken down or otherwise altered.

Oxidation, like inflammation, is part of our normal physiology. All of our body cells must carry out oxidation to stay alive. For example, oxidation is how our cells burn fuel to generate energy. Oxidation is also used by our defensive cells to break down pathogens and toxins. However, too much oxidation results in damage — which, in turn, can trigger inflammation. Oxidative stress has been associated with arthritis, cardiovascular disease, cancer, wrinkling of skin, hair loss, and graying of hair. Aging of the body is largely due to oxidative stress.

The body protects itself from oxidative stress by making powerful antioxidants. In addition, some vitamins, minerals, and other nutrients found in food, have antioxidant activity.

| Common Foods Rich in Antioxidants | |
|---|---|
| Fruits | Plums, strawberries, blueberries, blackberries, pomegranates, raspberries, grapes, watermelon, tomatoes, oranges |
| Vegetables | Kale, cabbage, cilantro, carrots, beets, sweet potatoes |
| Others | Green tea, dark chocolate, turmeric, garlic, cayenne pepper |

## Nitric Oxide

Nitric oxide is a free radical, but one that is very useful for the body. It is produced by our body cells and provides a number of vital functions. For example:

- As a potent free radical, nitric oxide is used by our immune system to destroy cancer cells, viruses, and bacteria.
- Nitric oxide dilates blood vessels, thus boosting local blood supply.
- Nitric oxide helps keep the inner lining of blood vessels soft and pliable – which is especially important for arteries.
- Nitric oxide promotes angiogenesis — production of new blood vessels.

Because of its effect on circulation and the immune system, nitric oxide has a profound effect on our health. Low levels of nitric oxide can contribute to reduced blood flow which in turn results in pain and degeneration. Many painful conditions are associated with poor blood supply. These conditions can improve by raising nitric oxide levels, as described in chapter 10.

In recent years, mainstream medicine has found many uses for nitric oxide as a therapeutic agent for a wide variety of health problems. It has been especially effective for pain relief. Can certain foods raise nitric oxide levels? Yes, here they are:

| Common Foods that Boost Nitric Oxide | |
|---|---|
| Fruits | Pomegranates, watermelon, citrus, cranberries |
| Vegetables | Spinach, kale, parsley, lettuce, celery, arugula, Swish chard, radishes, bok choy, fennel, endive, carrots, beets |
| Nuts & seeds | Walnuts, pistachios |
| Others | Sea food, dark chocolate, turmeric, garlic, cayenne pepper |

## Glutathione

Glutathione is the master detox molecule of the body. It is a broad-spectrum detoxifier and powerful antioxidant produced by our body cells. A glutathione molecule consists of three amino acids (glutamate, cysteine, and glycine) bonded together. Glutathione is especially important for liver function because this organ is the grand central station of cleansing and detox, as described in chapter 5.

Since toxicity and free radical damage are major contributors to aging and degeneration, optimal glutathione levels is an important key for health and healing. Food can have a profound effect on glutathione levels. In fact, the health promoting benefits of many foods may be at least partially attributed to their glutathione content or their ability to promote glutathione production in the body. For example, the foods listed in the table below are reputed to have health promoting properties. All of them promote higher glutathione levels in the body.

| Contain G'thione | | Promote G'thione Production |
|---|---|---|
| Asparagus | 28.3* | Broccoli |
| Avocado | 27.7 | Cauliflower |
| Spinach | 11.4 | Cabbage |
| Okra | 11.3 | Brussels sprouts |
| Broccoli | 9.1 | Garlic |
| Cantaloupe | 9.0 | Parsley |
| Tomato | 9.0 | Spinach |
| Carrot | 7.9 | Beets |
| Grapefruit | 7.9 | Turmeric |
| Orange | 7.3 | Cinnamon |
| Zucchini | 7.0 | Cardamom |
| Strawberry | 6.9 | Pomegranate |
| Watermelon | 6.6 | Whey |
| Papaya | 5.8 | Dandelion greens |
| Red bell pepper | 5.5 | Walnuts |
| Peach | 5.0 | Aloe vera |

(* Milligrams of glutathione per 100 grams of food.)

# Healing Foods

## Fruits

- **Apples** contain malic acid which helps remove toxic metals out of the body, stimulates cleansing of the liver, and can be beneficial for individuals with fibromyalgia and other forms of chronic pain. The skin of apples contains polyphenols which decrease colon cancer risk, inhibit aging of tissues, and promote stable blood sugar.
- **Bananas** are rich in potassium, help calm emotions and lift depression. Bananas contain phenols and carotenoids which have positive effects on human physiology. Bananas have traditionally been used in the treatment of various diseases.[3]
- **Blueberries, blackberries, and raspberries** are high in antioxidants. They are especially good for the heart, brain, and eyes. They are also rich in phytonutrients that have anticancer properties, as described in chapter 14.
- **Strawberries** are high in vitamin C and antioxidants. They also contain xylitol which may account for strawberries having a reputation for being good for teeth and gums.
- **Red or purple grapes** are high in antioxidants, especially resveratrol, which has been shown to promote cardiovascular health, and activates two so-called "anti-aging" genes.
- **Prunes** have very high antioxidant levels.
- **Pineapples** are high in vitamin C. They also contain bromelain, an enzyme that digests protein and has anti-inflammatory effects.
- **Papaya** are high in vitamin C and beta carotene. They also contain papain, a protein-digesting enzyme.
- **Watermelon** promotes cleansing of the intestines, liver, and kidneys. It is rich in lycopene and is reputed to be beneficial for individuals with psoriasis, arthritis, and kidney stones. It also promotes the production of nitric oxide which boosts microcirculation, protects the inner lining of blood vessels, and helps lower blood pressure.
- **Figs** are high in calcium and iron. They are also reputed to help dissolve mucus.
- **Pomegranates** are rich in antioxidants and help lower blood pressure. Human and animal studies suggest that it might reverse arterial plaquing.[4]
- **Kiwi fruit** are very rich in vitamin C. They also contain protein digesting enzymes, vitamin E, folate, and potassium Their high lutein content makes them especially beneficial for the eyes and brain.

# Vegetables

- **Asparagus** is a diuretic, anti-inflammatory, rich in glutathione.
- **Carrots** are rich in beta-carotene, which has many benefits, such as promoting eye health. Carrots also promote liver cleansing and contain oils that help eliminate intestinal parasites.
- **Beets** are rich in iron, promote cleansing of the liver and boost nitric oxide levels.
- **Dandelion greens** promote cleansing of the liver.
- **Celery** is an excellent source of minerals. It is soothing for the nervous system and helps to lower blood pressure.
- **Broccoli** has anticancer properties. It is rich in vitamin K and sulfur-containing oils which help detoxify the liver.
- **Kale** has the highest antioxidant levels of any vegetable. It is a good source of vitamin C, calcium, and iron. Like other dark green leafy vegetables, it promotes liver and blood cleansing. Like broccoli, it is rich in sulfur-containing oils.
- **Spinach**, like other dark green leafy vegetables, promotes cleansing of the liver and blood. It is also rich in antioxidants and iron.
- **Microgreens** are young seedlings of common food plants, such as wheat, barley, cilantro, peas, radishes, broccoli, and sunflower. The advantages of microgreens are as follows:
  - They may be grown at home, in small trays that have 2-3 inches of soil, and usually harvested within two weeks of planting.
  - Since they may be grown at home or purchased while still growing, they can be eaten shortly after harvesting — which means they provide the benefits of fresh vegetables straight from the garden.
  - They might contain up to 40 times higher levels of key nutrients, compared to the mature plant.
  - They are especially nutritious when grown in very fertile and mineral-rich soil, such as mushroom compost or worm castings.
  - All of the above features make microgreens ideal for helping the body recover from or prevent various illnesses. They offer strong anti-inflammatory and antioxidant protection, as well as having potentially therapeutic levels of various disease fighting phytonutrients. For example, microgreens are currently being investigated for their potential benefits in cancer treatment, as described in chapter 14.

## Nuts and Seeds

- **Walnuts** contain a wealth of nutrients that benefit the brain. They are rich in antioxidants, as well as promoting production of nitric oxide.
- **Flax seeds** are high in omega-3 oils, fiber, and phytonutrients. They promote intestinal motility and enhance the growth of beneficial bacteria.
- **Chia seeds** are often called a "superfood," because they bring together a number of valuable elements. They are high in omega-3 oils, and rich in minerals, soluble fiber, and antioxidants. They tend to have an almost immediate energizing effect and therefore provide an alternative to coffee and other stimulants.
- **Pumpkin seeds** are rich in zinc and protein. They are good for the prostate, as well as containing oils that help expel worms.[5]
- **Sesame seeds** are rich in minerals. The lignins in sesame seeds have many health benefits, such as protecting DNA from free radical damage. They also help lower cholesterol and reduce inflammation.[6]
- **Almonds** have long been reputed to have anticancer properties, which is now supported studies.[7]

## Specialty Foods

The following foods are reputed to be helpful for individuals trying to resolve various health issues and improve health.

- **Noni.** Promotes emotional stability, reduces allergic reactions, lowers blood pressure and cholesterol levels, and stabilizes blood sugar. Helps to cleanse and heal the digestive and respiratory systems. Beneficial for the immune system, helps resolve strep throat and sinus infections, eliminates yeast, fungus, and parasites. Helps improve microcirculation by elevating nitric oxide levels.
- **Aloe Vera.** In ancient Egypt, aloe vera was known as the plant of immortality. It has been used for thousands of years throughout the world for its many health benefits. It optimizes absorption and utilization of nutrients by the body, activates macrophages and T cells, and promotes higher levels of stem cells. It gives a powerful boost to the immune system, reduces allergic and autoimmune reactions, relieves inflammation, helps balance blood sugar, and promotes regeneration, especially of the digestive system and skin.
- **Acai Berries**: Excellent nutritive tonic for someone who is depleted or recovering from illness. Rich in antioxidants, as well as easily absorbed protein and beneficial fats.

- **Goji Berries** elevate mood. In China, goji is known as the "Happy Berry." They have strong antioxidant properties, promote physical regeneration, healthy eyes and vision, strong immune system, and healthy libido.
- **Colostrum** is the milk-like liquid produced by the mammary glands of pregnant mammals just prior to giving birth. Colostrum is a cocktail of easily absorbed fats, protein, sugars, and other substances that support the immune system and promote growth. This is a perfect first food for the newborn's underdeveloped digestive system and immune system. For similar reasons, it can be helpful for individuals with digestive and immune system problems, such as frequent respiratory infections, allergies, and leaky gut syndrome.

# Chapter 4
# Food as Medicine
## Part 2 – The Principles

Do No Harm
Let the Body Heal Itself
The Triangle of Health
Food as Medicine in a Nutshell

*"The best way to fight a war is to not fight it at all."*
*– Sun Tzu*

The best way to treat disease is to not get sick in the first place. Maintaining health is ultimately easier and requires less time and money than restoring health. Stated differently, to the extent that we do not spend time and money to stay healthy, we will probably have to spend more time and more money to regain our health. This is reason alone to focus on wellness and practice prevention. Furthermore, the health that we do recover after illness may not match the health we had originally. For example, by relying on fast and cheap processed foods that clog the colon and overload the liver, we might be setting the stage for the need to remove the gall bladder, after which digestive functions may be compromised.[1]

High quality whole food is our best resource for maintaining optimum health. When the body does get sick, look first to the same whole foods as your medicine. We may not even have to make any special adjustments – other than simply adopting a wholesome diet that the body perhaps needed all along.

Hippocrates' strong emphasis on the use of food to maintain and restore health goes hand in hand with another one of his famous principles which is the foundation of the Hippocratic Oath taken by medical doctors: "Above all else, do no harm."

The principle of doing no harm is not just for health-care practitioners. It is also important for anyone endeavoring to restore or otherwise improve their own health by using everyday foods or other nutritional products.

# Do No Harm

The idea of doing no harm seems so obvious that we might overlook it. Yet, Hippocrates saw fit to call attention to it — which should give us a clue that it might not be as easy as it seems. Below are the specifics on how to do no harm in our quest for vibrant health.

- Let everyday foods be your first medicine of choice.
- Beware of short-term gain followed by long-term loss.
- Treat the cause of the illness, rather than symptoms.
- Therapeutic diet vs maintenance diet: know the difference.

## Food First

Everyday foods and other nutritional products, used properly, are usually the safest and often most effective way of resolving a given health issue. Here are the basic ways we can use food and other nutritional products as medicine:

- We select foods that provide higher levels of certain nutrients to help resolve a given health issue. For example, we might favor foods that are rich in vitamin C, so as to help the body fight off an infection or promote healing of an injured tissues.
- We select foods known to have special properties beyond the usual nutrients. For example, if we sprain an ankle, we might gravitate toward pineapple because it has the enzyme, bromelain, which helps reduce inflammation.
- We can use food extracts or supplements that have even higher levels of substances which are relevant for addressing the illness in question. For example, we might take very large amounts of vitamin C to help reduce inflammation and pain.

The last bullet point above calls attention to the fact that nutrients which help maintain normal physiology when consumed in concentrations found in whole foods, can have other therapeutic effects when used in larger concentrations. For example, vitamin C in whole foods has many regulatory functions. Beyond that, some health practitioners use large doses of vitamin C, sometimes intravenously, to treat serious pathologies. However, care must to be taken to assure that the high doses do not create more problems than they resolve, as described below.

## When Medicine Becomes Poison

This is a good time to remember the distinction between the purely nutritional effect of a given food or nutritional supplement and its medicinal effect. As described on page 23, using food as food means that our goal is to *maintain* health, while using food as medicine means that our goal is to *restore* health.

Stated differently, using food as food means that we provide the body with all nutrients needed to *maintain* normal and healthy physiology. Using food or supplements as medicine means we are using the same nutrients to *change* our physiology — hopefully for the better.

Admittedly, the line between a purely nutritional effect and a medicinal effect may be blurred in many instances. However, the distinction between the two is still important if we wish to use any product safely and effectively. Here is the reason: Anything that can change our physiology for the better can also change it for the worse if used excessively or improperly.

When we understand the distinction between the purely nutritive function of any product and its possible medicinal function, we are less likely to misuse it, and more likely to use it safely and effectively. We understand that an otherwise essential nutrient can easily become problematical if removed from its supportive whole food matrix and concentrated to high levels that the body normally does not encounter. For example, the minerals zinc, iron, and selenium each serve a number of normal regulatory functions but can become toxic in higher concentrations.

If a given diet is based on a wide variety of quality whole foods, we can easily get all the minerals we need to meet the body's needs. Under such circumstances, the chances of toxicity due to excess is virtually zero. However, iron, zinc, selenium, and many other minerals can reach toxic levels if taken in amounts that exceed the levels we encounter in whole foods. This can easily happen when we ingest these minerals in the form of supplements. The same can happen with vitamins, especially the fat-soluble vitamins, such as vitamin A. In other words, the likelihood of creating toxicity increases with the increased use of nutrients which have been removed from their whole matrix.

## Short-Term Gain and Long-Term Loss

When we think in terms of short-term gain, we are likely to become short-sighted. When we become short-sighted, we become vulnerable to long-term loss. One way of preventing short-sightedness is to address a given problem at its source, rather than focusing too much on getting rid of immediate symptoms.

A common way that health-conscious individuals try to resolve a given health issue is to take one or more isolated nutrients or herbs. The kitchen cabinet or refrigerator of health seeking individuals might be filled with bottles and packages of pills, capsules, powders, and liquids containing vitamins, minerals, herbs, or combinations thereof. Though they might all be potentially useful, there are several potential problems with this approach:

- As previously mentioned, we can unbalance ourselves nutritionally by relying too heavily on isolated nutrients, rather than whole foods. The long-term consequences may not be obvious, but imbalances can gradually accumulate when we regularly take large amounts of nutrients that have been separated from their whole-food matrix and concentrated to very high levels.

- The body can be exposed binders, fillers, preservatives, stabilizers, artificial flavoring, and artificial colors which are frequently used to make supplements.

- The body can be exposed to other substances that do not appear on the label, such as chemical residue from the manufacturing process, or aluminum and plastics from packaging. Granted, the amount of such residue in a given dose might be negligibly small. However, the effects of such chemical residue are multiplied when we take many supplements for an extended period of time.

- Deficiencies may occur. We might ingest large amounts of a specialty food for its therapeutic value, and unknowingly marginalize other foods that contain needed nutrients.

- Unwanted weight gain may occur. If we introduce a calorically dense food extract, such as coconut oil, but do not decrease the calorically dense foods.

## Treating the Cause

Here are three signs that a given remedy is not correcting the cause of a given health challenge:

- We have to continue taking it indefinitely to experience relief.
- The remedy becomes less effective over time.
- We develop harmful side effects.

Again, we are less likely to do long-term harm if we endeavor to resolve a given health issue at its source rather than just targeting the symptoms. However, this is easier said than done, because the cause is often not obvious, or perhaps not as simple as a deficiency of a single nutrient.

Typically, when we use nutritional products to resolve a given health issue, we are just guessing at its cause and hope that our remedy of choice will do the trick. For example, if we feel tired and stressed out, we might take B vitamins. Similarly, we might try to resolve joint pain with anti-inflammatory herbs and supplements. This approach is not very precise, but health-conscious individuals might facetiously justify it by saying that such an approach still makes more sense than other strategies that seem to regard joint pain as a deficiency of Tylenol; or clogged arteries as a deficiency of statin drugs. Tongue-in-cheek aside, I am inclined to agree. However, we can do better.

## We can Do Better

I have occasionally encountered patients and students who reported that they started feeling better when they stopped taking all their medication and supplements. I'm not suggesting here to avoid such products, but rather to use them conservatively and judiciously. Using herbs and supplements conservatively and judiciously means that we first focus on restoring as much of our health as we can by using the same resources that keep us healthy in the first place — nutritious food, clean water, exercise, fresh air, sunshine, and adequate rest.

In other words, even if we use herbs and supplements to help us get well, we should also contemplate why we got sick in the first place. In particular, we should think of the specific steps we can take to optimize our use of everyday foods as medicine. The first step in doing this is to understand the distinction between a therapeutic diet and a maintenance diet.

## Therapeutic Diet and Maintenance Diet

A maintenance diet is used indefinitely. A therapeutic diet is used for a certain period of time to help achieve a specific health goal, such as losing weight.

The distinction between the two is important because a diet that works well initially to help achieve a specific health goal is not necessarily sustainable in the long-run. It could, perhaps gradually, become problematical down the road. In other words, it can produce short-term gain and long-term loss. For example, weight reduction is a common reason that many individuals change their diet. Rapid weight loss is often achieved by going on a high protein diet. However, the same approach done long-term can insidiously harm the body in a number of ways, such as damaging the kidneys and accelerating the aging of tissues.[2,3] This is why dietitians and doctors that use high protein diets to helps resolve a particular health problem will monitor the patient carefully and limit the time period for the diet.

In other words, we do not assume that a diet that produces good short-term results will continue to produce good long-term results. We can avoid such pitfalls by first simply asking ourselves whether our intention is to follow a given eating plan as a short-term therapeutic measure to resolve a specific health issue, or as a long-term maintenance diet.

What if you are not sure? What if it's a little bit of both? Either way, it's okay; you just have to be attentive to your inner signals, so you can make adjustments as needed. Be attentive to the changing needs of the body, rather than feeling obligated to strictly adhere to a certain dietary doctrine.

Regarding the ideal maintenance diet, a good rule of thumb is to select foods that provide all needed nutrients in the cleanest and most digestible form possible. Regarding the ideal therapeutic diet, the rule of thumb is essentially the same, except that the proportion of different foods might be tweaked a bit to address the specific health goal of the moment.

On the bright side, with a therapeutic diet, the health challenges we are facing will probably motivate us to do the diet more methodically than our everyday maintenance diet. This alone can greatly increase our chances of success.

> We can use food as medicine safely and effectively by first understanding the distinction between a therapeutic diet and a maintenance diet.

# Let the Body Heal Itself

In terms of practical application, letting the body heal itself means two things:

- The health-care practitioner favors modalities which engage the body's capacity for self-healing.
- The practitioner favors the safest, least invasive, and most conservative treatment to resolve the problem at hand. In that regard, letting the body heal itself is an extension of the principle of doing no harm.

Happily, the safest and most conservative modalities also tend to be the best at engaging the body's capacity for self-healing. Why? Quite simply, gentle methods are more likely to activate the parasympathetic nervous system — which essentially puts the body into a restorative and regenerative mode.

In contrast, the more invasive therapeutic modalities are more likely to trigger the sympathetic nervous system which, in turn, triggers the release of stress hormones. Massive sympathetic dominance is called the fight-or-flight response, in which the body has no time to rest and heal because it is in crisis mode.

When the body is in sympathetic dominance, it is just trying to survive, so it uses up energy quickly and often inefficiently, thereby depleting its resources and creating toxicity.[4] When the body is in sympathetic dominance, it is definitely not in regeneration mode; it is in degeneration mode.

Since the sympathetic system is not conducive to healing, why would we be tempted to use invasive methods that provoke sympathetic response? The usual reason is expediency. Such methods tend to produce fast results. Therefore, if we are in a lot of pain, we might get a cortisone shot or use other strong medication. Similarly, if allergies prevent us from doing our work, we might take antihistamines to dry up sinuses. These fast methods can be a blessing during a crisis but are likely to undermine health if used regularly. Cortisone and other pain medication, used habitually, tend to disrupt the body's capacity to regenerate.[5,6] The ideal healing strategy is one that helps relieve suffering as quickly as possible, while also allowing the body to relax and regenerate.

**Use the most conservative treatment first**

- Before you start taking things to resolve a health issue, see if you can simply stop doing whatever is causing or aggravating the problem. For instance, before you take a drug for insomnia, see if you can remove the cause of the insomnia – stop listening to the news or watching violent movies before bedtime.
- Many commonly encountered health issues are either caused or aggravated by too many calories and not enough vitamins, minerals, phytonutrients, and fiber. In other words, too much building foods, not enough cleaning foods; too much bread, pasta, meat, and extracted oils, and not enough fresh produce. Therefore, a simple way of using food as medicine is to *decrease the high calorie foods and increase fresh produce.*
- After you have done as much as you can with everyday foods, exercise, and elimination of stressors, the next step is to explore other methods, such as herbs and nutritional supplements, acupuncture, massage, and chiropractic. Favor first the safest and most conservative treatments before resorting to more invasive modalities.
- Take the minimum amount of any medicinal substance to achieve the desired result.
- Don't take a product or apply a therapy longer than needed. The more invasive the procedure, or toxic the substance, the more quickly you want to stop using it.

**Let the Body Rest**

The simplest way to let the body heal itself is to just let it rest. This principle is strongly promoted by Natural Hygiene, which is an integrated system of healing and healthy living. In addressing specific health challenges, Natural Hygiene endeavors to fully engage the body's own self-healing capacity through fasting, rest, proper exercise, clean water, clean air, and sunshine.

In our urgency, we tend to marginalize these great natural healers. Fortunately, science is gradually validating the healing power of these simple and natural remedies. For example, the right kind of food, exercise, sunshine, and fasting all raise nitric oxide levels. Beyond that, letting the body rest essentially allows it to "reboot" itself.

## Rebooting the System

When animals in the wild become ill, they often abstain from food. In so doing, the body does not merely clean up the back-log of waste. Healing and regeneration are accelerated. The body seems to restore or rebalance itself on many levels, like a computer that is rebooted to an earlier state of greater functionality.

Letting the body physiologically rest is an ancient principle for healing, which is now being validated by modern science. For example, research indicates that oxidative stress decreases and nitric oxide levels increase during a fast.[7] Fasting and caloric restriction have also been shown to alter gene expression in a way that essentially allows the body to age more slowly.[8]

Our physiology is regulated by countless neurological reflexes and hormonal feedback loops which maintain proper blood sugar, blood pressure, cholesterol and triglycerides levels, digestion, respiration, heart rate, and hormones. All these can be disrupted by toxicity, deficiencies, and other stressors. And all of them can improve by just giving the body some down-time.

> By temporarily abstaining from food or reducing it, the body can restore itself like a computer that is rebooted to an earlier state.

## The Fast Way to Heal

Total abstinence from food for extended periods might be difficult or not advisable for some individuals. The good news is that once we understand the basic principle behind fasting – letting the body rest – we can easily apply it without necessarily abstaining from all food for days at a time. Here are three options for giving the body a physiological rest while still eating everyday:

- Reducing total calories
- Increasing the proportion of cleansing foods
- Intermittent fasting

## Hard reboot and soft reboot

A long water fast may be compared to a total reboot of a computer. A total reboot is a rather lengthy process that wipes out all programs except for those provided by the manufacturer. In contrast, intermittent fasting, caloric reduction or increasing the proportion of cleansing foods, may be likened to a soft reboot, wherein the computer is restored to an earlier state that predates the start of the problem.

The gentler methods may not produce the deep results of an extended water fast but tend to be more doable, as well as providing other options in situations where a long water fast is not advisable.

Even without fasting per se', the simple act of reducing calories allows the body to catch-up on needed cleansing and repair. In fact, since the individual does not totally abstain from food, he or she can stay on the program longer and thus receive most of the benefits of a water fast. A common way to do this is to drink freshly squeezed vegetable or fruit juice for a certain period of time.

The problem with reducing calories by just drinking juices is that it can leave us feeling hungry and dissatisfied because caloric content is one of the major factors that allows us to feel satisfied with a given meal. The other factor that makes us feel satisfied is the presence of bulk the in stomach. Juices are low in calories and also low in bulk. The solution is to apply the second principle: eat more cleansing foods — the whole food, rather than just drinking the juice.

Cleansing foods are low in calories, while providing higher levels of fiber, water, vitamins, minerals, and phytonutrients. All of these combine to allow us to feel satisfied on fewer calories, while also giving the body the nutritional resources it needs to cleanse and repair. One application of this principle is to eat one type of juicy fruit, such as grapes, watermelon or oranges for a given period of time.[9,10]

An even gentler method is to just increase the consumption of fresh and raw produce without necessarily eliminating other high-calorie foods, such as bread, potatoes, and meat. Ideally, the high-calorie foods will decrease with little or no effort simply by focusing on increasing the fresh produce. One advantage of this method is that we need not be concerned about time restriction; we just do it for long as it feels right.

Eating more fruit can be as simple as eating more fruit. Typically, fruit can be consumed with virtually no preparation. You just reach into the fruit bowl, pick up an apple and eat it.

Eating more vegetables generally does take preparation. One way to increase veggies is by making delicious fruit and vegetable smoothies, such as baby spinach blended with blueberries.

## Intermittent Fasting

Intermittent fasting seems to provide many of the benefits of prolonged caloric restriction.[11] Intermittent fasting can be as simple as delaying the first meal of the day. This gives the body more time to cleanse and heal. How long should we wait? As long as it feels right. In other words, *just wait until you're good and hungry, rather than just eating out of habit.*

The ideal way to fast is what the Natural Hygienists call "biological fasting," in which the individual fasts only when true hunger is not present; and the fast is ended when true hunger returns. This might seem simplistic and naïve, until we take the time to understand the concept of *true* hunger.

As suggested above, we often eat out of habit. Or, we eat as a way of coping with stress. We are taught at an early age to eat according to the outer clock, rather than our inner signals. Watching television seems to promote eating – especially chips and other fast-foods. True hunger is beyond all that. The point here is that we can apply the principle of biological fasting by simply abstaining from food until we are genuinely hungry.

The body can cleanse and repair very nicely when we give it 12 hours of daily rest from food. Unless there is a medical need to eat more frequently, most individuals can do a daily 12-hour fast with little or no effort. It is as simple as not eating late at night, and then abstaining from food the following morning until true hunger emerges. For added cleansing and regeneration, we can intentionally extend the fast beyond 12 hours if it feels right.

On most days, my inclination is to give my body about 14 hours of rest from food. Occasionally, I might go 16 hours or longer. I usually do not plan on the longer periods. I simply wait to eat until I'm hungry, rather than absentmindedly eating just because it's noon. On the days that I delay my first meal beyond 1pm, my body feels light and energized, and my mind is clear and sharp.

If a 16 hour fast seems like too long for you, it probably is. The point here is to pay attention when you awaken in the morning. Pay attention to the inner voice that might be whispering to you to wait a little longer before you "break the fast."

> We can apply the principle of biological fasting by simply abstaining from food until we are genuinely hungry.

51

## A Faster Way to Fast

For those who have done several water-fasts and feel comfortable doing so, another option is to also abstain from water. This is called "dry-fasting." Not surprisingly, dry fasting is not done for an extended period time; two or three days are typical. Dry fasting more than seven days is not generally recommended. Here are some of the reported benefits of dry fasting:

- According to some testimonials, a short dry fast might be easier than a long water fast, while providing equal or better results. I found this to be true for me.
- A dry fast supposedly burns fat faster than a water fast.
- A dry fast is said to cleanse the body more deeply and rapidly than a water fast of the same duration.
- A dry fast is said to destroy pathogens and break down diseased tissues more quickly than a water fast.
- A dry fast is said to balance and calm the mind more effectively than a water fast. Interestingly enough, when the prophets and monks of ancient times fasted, they typically did a dry fast.

## Do it Properly

Fasting should be done with thoughtfulness and care. As with other potentially powerful therapeutic tools, fasting can do more harm than good if used excessively or improperly.

Fasting for more than a week or so should be done under proper supervision, at least for beginners. The longer the fast, the more thoroughly the individual should prepare himself or herself physically, mentally, and emotionally. This is where the guidance of someone experienced in fasting can be most helpful.

How long can a human being safely fast? Some individuals have fasted for 30 days or longer and report healing of issues that were not responding to anything else. Obviously, this is not for everyone! As we might expect, those who have more body-fat can fast for longer periods of time compared to thinner individuals. However, even for those who feel up to it, fasting for such a long time is best done at a fasting facility, supported by a trained staff which includes medical personnel who monitor the individual's vital signs, blood, and urine.[12]

# The Triangle of Health

In order to properly use nutrition for healing, we must recognize that it is part of a bigger picture. This bigger picture may be visualized as a triangle.

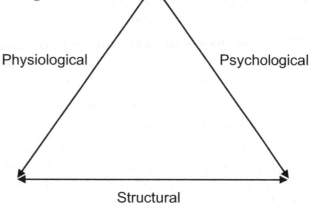

The psychological side refers to our thoughts and emotions. The structural side refers to the physical frame of the body. The physiological side refers to the biochemical workings of the body. We care for the psychological side through mindfulness, meditation, and choosing our thoughts, words, and actions. We care for the physical side with exercise, as well as hands-on methods of healing, such as massage, chiropractic, and osteopathy. We care for the physiological side with high quality food and perhaps supplements and medicinal herbs.

The three sides have equal length, reminding us of their equal importance. Each side is depicted as a bidirectional arrow which converges with the other two, reminding us that the three are interrelated and interdependent. They complement one another, but they cannot replace each other. This means we would not neglect one side and expect to take up the slack by giving more attention to the other two. For example, we would not expect to use nutritional means to correct a health problem which arises from lack of exercise or emotional stress. By maintaining such mindfulness and acting accordingly, we are able to make the best possible use of food as medicine, because the nutritional side of our triangle is well supported by the other two.

# Food as Medicine in a Nut Shell

- **Let the body heal itself**. Favor therapeutic measures that engage or cooperate with the body's capacity for self-healing, rather than disrupting it. These methods tend to be the safest and least invasive.

- **Allow the body to rest and reboot** through fasting or reduction of high-calorie foods. This is the simplest and safest way to allow the body to heal itself.

- Be mindful of the distinction between a **therapeutic diet and a maintenance diet.**

- **Focus on the cause**, rather than symptoms. The cause generally involves a disruption of the body's capacity for self-healing. This doesn't mean we ignore the symptoms; it simply means we look for ways of removing symptoms by resolving their root cause.

- **Remember the triangle.** Food is most effective as medicine when an unbalanced diet is the primary stressor that overpowers the body's capacity for self-healing. When diet is not the primary stressor, food can still be helpful, but we must also address the primary issues, which often involve lack of exercise, lack of rest, or emotional stress.

The chapters that follow will apply the above principles to facilitate recovery from many common health problems, ranging from minor ailments to serious diseases. For most everyday health challenges, such as unwanted weight gain and indigestion, the use of food as medicine can be as simple as selecting the cleanest and most nutritious food that we can find, and occasionally allowing the body to rest from the usual foods. Yes, it can be that simple.

To apply these same principles to serious health challenges, our next step is to deepen our understanding of how the body digests food and cleans itself of waste products. These topics are addressed in the two chapters that follow.

# Chapter 5
# Healing by Cleansing

Backlog
Portals of Elimination
Start with the Gut
Cleaning out the Filters
The One Day Cleanse

*"When you're green inside, you're clean inside."*
*−Bernard Jenson N.D.*

In previous centuries, internal cleansing was often used to support recovery from illness. However, since the early-20th century, its therapeutic role has been marginalized and sometimes ridiculed or attacked by mainstream medicine.[1,2.]

Some critics do not necessarily dismiss the idea that toxicity contributes to illness; they simply see no value in doing anything about it, beyond healthy food and exercise. In principle, I am inclined to agree. However, these critics do not consider an important point: food is often not fully digested and the residue not fully eliminated from one meal to the next. Digestion and cleanup are often inhibited by constitutional weaknesses, sedentary lifestyle, emotional unrest, or other stressors. Have you ever "tasted" food or smelled it in your armpits the day after eating it? Or two days perhaps? In other words, the body has to process one meal while it is still dealing with the previous one. Over time, the result is a backlog of unfinished business.

## Backlog

The backlog consists of accumulated debris which the body stores wherever it can, such as fat tissue. Of equal importance, there is also a backlog of repair and regeneration which the body has not been able to complete because resources are limited and there is just so much that can be accomplished on any given day.

Modern science has been gradually validating the ancient practice of promoting internal cleansing to support healing from illness. We have no shortage of studies linking toxicity to various diseases. For example, some of the putrefactive bi-products of intestinal bacteria are rather potent carcinogens.[3,4] Some of them produce the foul smell of feces and have been linked to colorectal cancer.[5,6,7,8] For these reasons, more and more medical practitioners, including some gastroenterologists, are recognizing the value of supporting the body's ability to cleanse itself.[9,10,11]

# Portals of Elimination

To appreciate the need for internal cleansing, we need only consider the large amount of anatomical hardware and physiological software which are dedicated to cleansing. Here are the main portals through which the body eliminates waste:

- Large intestine
- Liver
- Gall bladder
- Kidneys
- Lungs
- Skin

These organs are supported by literally thousands of miles of blood and lymph vessels. Since the body obviously gives high priority to internal cleansing, it should serve to remind us to cooperate with the body's cleansing activities. Our cooperation begins by increasing the proportion of cleansing foods, as described in the previous chapter. In fact, this is frequently the only step we need to take.

### Increase Cleansing Foods

Your ideal diet provides a balance of building foods and cleansing foods, as described in chapter 3. Therefore, our cooperation can simply take the form of temporarily increasing the proportion of cleansing foods, which means that we also decrease the building foods. In other words, we increase foods that feature higher levels of fiber, water, vitamins, minerals, and phytonutrients, while decreasing high-calorie foods. This means we increase fruits and vegetables, while decreasing animal products, grains, dry beans, nuts, and seeds.

If you the cleansing plan described above is to your liking, you might settle into a routine of doing it periodically. However, if you feel inclined to explore options for deeper cleansing, the next step is to gain a deeper understanding of the sources of toxicity.

**Sources of Toxicity**

The main sources of toxicity are:

- toxins taken into the body through food, water, and air.
- metabolic waste generated by our body cells.
- metabolic waste generated by microbes living in the body, most notably the gut.

The latter point is major. To the extent that digestion and absorption are compromised, food lingering in the digestive tract provides food for bacteria and other microbes. Some of the microbes produce beneficial substances, but others produce toxins, including some potent carcinogens. This is why internal cleansing should begin with the gut.

# Start with the Gut

The large intestine is the dirtiest place in the body. This is significant because toxins from the large intestine can be absorbed into the blood, contributing to a wide variety of degenerative conditions, including cancer and arthritis.[12]

A clean large intestine starts with a bowel movement at least once a day and preferably more. Yet, some folks evacuate their bowels every 2-3 days or longer and consider it normal. We must also bear in mind that the gut is made of living tissue that has to be able to rest and regenerate. Just as debris can accumulate, so can the effects of wear and tear on living tissue. Hemorrhoids from having to strain at every bowel movement is one of many health problems that can result from chronic constipation.

The foundation for maintaining a clean gut is to include enough plant fiber and water to allow for at least one bowel movement per day. Yes, it is that simple. However, when the gut has been compromised by years of constipating foods and antibiotics, we may need to take other measures to restore the gut to a state of health, as described in the next chapter. For now, let us consider how body normally filters out the toxins which enter the blood from the gut and our body cells.

# Cleaning Out the Filters

Nutrients and toxins that enter the blood from the intestines go straight to the liver. The liver devotes a lot of its energy and resources to detoxing and cleansing the entire body. Therefore, after the large intestine has been allowed to cleanse itself, the individual can give some attention to the liver. Many health issues, such as hemorrhoids, can improve when the liver is allowed to cleanse itself.

## Cleansing the Liver

- In the morning, drink the juice of one lemon in warm water.
- Increase dark green leafy vegetables, such as fresh dandelion.
- Increase cruciferous vegetables, such as kale, broccoli, and Brussels sprouts.
- Drink apple juice. Use organic juice because conventionally grown apples are usually sprayed heavily with pesticides and fungicides.
- Drink carrot and beet juice — about 4 parts carrots to 1part beets. These two vegetables support the liver in a number of ways, such as encouraging the production of glutathione, a potent cellular cleanser as described in chapter 3.

## Cleansing the Kidneys

The kidneys, like the liver, filter the blood. How do they differ? The liver has the capacity to remove large molecules that do not dissolve well in water, whereas the kidneys remove small, water-soluble molecules. In other words, as a filter, the kidney is finer and more delicate than the liver. The kidneys are more easily damaged by physical or chemical irritants. Therefore, one of the indirect benefits of keeping the large intestine and liver clean and in good working order, is that we can avoid subjecting the kidneys to large molecules or other irritants that would otherwise contribute to ageing and degeneration of the kidneys.

The simplest and safest way of directly helping the kidneys is to drink ample amounts of clean water, while increasing consumption of juicy fruits and vegetables, such as watermelon and cucumbers. In addition, individuals who have kidney problems are advised to avoid overconsuming protein, especially in the form of meat and glutinous grains.

## Cleansing the Lungs and Skin

We think of the lungs as being vital for bringing oxygen into the body. However, they are also important for eliminating carbon dioxide and other metabolic waste. Elimination through the skin is also important. One pound of waste may be discharged though the skin every day.

The lungs and skin generally eliminate molecules that are small and water-soluble. However, when the large intestine and liver become overloaded, the lungs and skin must work harder and eliminate molecules that are bigger and less water soluble.

Here are some ways to promote lung and skin cleansing:
- Deep breathing and exercise.
- Dry skin brushing. Use a loofa, coarse brush, or rough towel.
- Alternating hot (3 minutes) and cold (30 seconds) showers to stimulate circulation through the skin. As a point of caution, individuals with a heart condition should consult with their physician before using this method.
- Induce sweating through vigorous exercise or in a sauna. (Individuals with a heart condition should consult with their physician first).

## Shaking Out the Filters

Just as the air filter in your car needs to be periodically shaken and cleaned, our own internal filters also require physical activity to allow them to properly cleanse and maintain themselves. One common reason that a given diet "doesn't work" for a given individual might be that he or she is seeking a dietary solution to a problem stemming from a lack of exercise.

Furthermore, unlike the oil filter or air filter in your car, the liver, kidneys, lungs, and skin are not mechanical devices that are easily replaced. They are made of delicate living tissue that require the right nutrition to repair and regenerate themselves.

Physical exercise promotes cleansing through all portals of elimination. It also promotes proper nourishment of these organs. Exercise also promotes good digestion, enhances the immune system, elevates emotions, reduces food cravings, and stabilizes blood sugar and blood pressure.

# The One Day Cleanse

This cleansing plan can be done for one or more days. If you find it is beneficial, you can do it once a week, every other week, or once a month. This plan is even more effective if you also exercise outdoors during the day, especially in the morning before breakfast.

## Morning

After your brisk morning exercise, you can use any of the following options for breakfast:

- Just drink water until lunch time (unless you have blood sugar issues).
- Freshly squeezed vegetable juice.
- A mono-fruit meal consisting of one type of fresh fruit.
- A smoothie made of green leafy vegetables, water, and enough fresh fruit to make it tasty.

## Afternoon

- A green smoothie made of the fruits and vegetables of your choice.
- A fruit mono-meal.
- A raw vegetable salad. Use a low-fat dressing consisting of any combination of the following: lemon juice, orange juice, blended tomato, mango or strawberries, chunks of soaked sun-dried tomatoes.
- Fruit followed by a vegetable salad.
- If you get hungry between lunch and dinner, have fresh fruit or a green smoothie.

## Evening

- For dinner, you can use the same basic options as lunch, perhaps with a different combination of ingredients.
- The same fruits and vegetables used to make the salad dressing can also be rearranged into a delicious raw soup, which can replace or complement the salad.
- If you get hungry after dinner, you can have a fruit snack.

# Chapter 6
# Healthy Gut

Digestion
Gut Problems
Leaky Gut Syndrome
Food Combining
Gut Healing Diets
Tips for Digestive Health

*"All disease begins in the gut."*
*—Hippocrates*

Of all body systems, the digestive system is the one that is most obviously affected by food. Diarrhea, constipation, hemorrhoids, gas, bloating, ulcers, acid reflux, colitis, colon cancer, gall stones, etc., can all be caused or aggravated by the wrong diet and can be greatly improved or reversed with the right diet. What's more, science is validating the ancient idea that a dirty and weakened digestive system can lead to many other health problems.

To make the best possible use of food for resolving gut issues, let us first look at how digestion works.

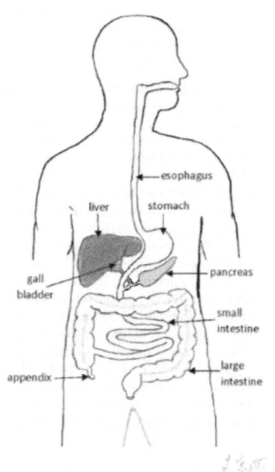

# Digestion

Digestion is the extraction of nutrients from food. This is done within the digestive tract, also known as the gut.

The gut is a tube which starts with the mouth and ends with the anus. It is about 30 feet long. As food is digested in the gut, the liberated nutrients are absorbed into the blood. Nutrients and residue that do not pass into the blood continue on to the large intestine and are eventually expelled as feces. The bulk of the large intestine is called the colon, therefore the two terms are often used interchangeably.

## Acidophilus and Friends

The key to a healthy gut is a thriving population of intestinal microorganisms, most notably bacteria. In addition to bacteria, the other beasties of the bowels include yeast, protozoa (such as amebae) and worms.

Digestion of food and absorption of nutrients require the right kind of intestinal bacteria. For convenience, bacteria may be placed into two broad categories. They are putrefactive bacteria and fermentative bacteria.

- **Putrefactive bacteria** include Escherichia coli (E. coli) and other microbes which feed mostly on protein, producing toxic byproducts.[1] These bacteria also feed on bile salts, which are produced by the liver. Bile salts help to digest fat. Therefore, the liver produces more bile salts in response to larger amounts of fat in the diet.

  Putrefactive bacteria account for some of the toxicity associated with overconsuming high-protein foods. These toxins include hydrogen sulfide (a gas that smells like rotten eggs) and other foul-smelling metabolic poisons that contribute to colon cancer and other bowel problems.[2,3,4]

  Not surprisingly, carnivorous animals have a much shorter digestive tract compared to omnivores and herbivores. Meat consists largely of concentrated fat and protein – a potential feast for putrefactive bacteria. Therefore, carnivores have to evacuate their bowels as quickly as possible.

  The human digestive tract is longer than that of carnivores, and not nearly as efficient at digesting meat. Large amounts of meat in our intestines can be a problem, especially if the individual is chronically constipated. Under such conditions, the body is subjected to constant low-grade toxicity from the putrefactive bi-products seeping into the blood. This is why plant fiber is a vital part of a healthy diet; it speeds up transit time and absorbs toxins. Plant fiber also provides food for beneficial bacteria, also known as fermentative bacteria.

- **Fermentative bacteria** break down plant fiber and other carbohydrates, producing many useful byproducts. Here are the health benefits of fermentative bacteria:
  - They produce vitamins, including vitamin K, folic acid, biotin, and vitamin $B_{12}$.[5]
  - They produce short-chain fatty acids that nourish the cells of the intestinal lining.
  - They promote mineral absorption.
  - They produce digestive enzymes.
  - Some of their biproducts are absorbed into the blood and support the immune system.
  - Their byproducts reduce inflammation and allergic reactions.
  - They produce lactic acid, which discourages the growth of putrefactive bacteria, yeast, and larger parasites, such as round worms, flukes, and tapeworms. All these organisms produce noxious chemicals that usher in other gut problems.

# Gut Problems

Constipation, bloating, and gas are so common that most folks either ignore these issues or regard them as normal. However, these conditions are not merely a hindrance to socializing; they are the visible (and sometimes audible) expressions of hidden imbalances that eventually lead to more serious problems. Here are a few examples.

- Hemorrhoids consist of inflamed and swollen veins in the wall of the anus.

- Peptic ulcers consist of erosion of the inner lining of the stomach or first part of the small intestine.

- Irritable bowel syndrome (IBS) is irritation anywhere along the gut, due to stress. Symptoms include pain, cramping, nausea, loss of appetite, diarrhea, constipation, flatulence, and mucus in the stool. If it occurs entirely in the colon, the condition is also called spastic colon or irritable colon.

- Inflammatory bowel disease (IBD) is inflammation along the GI tract. One form is called ulcerative colitis, which involves chronic inflammation and bleeding of the inner lining of the large intestine. The other form is called Crohn's disease, which involves inflammation anywhere along the gut, from the stomach to the rectum.

- Diverticulosis is an out-pocketing of the wall of the large intestine. The individual may have no symptoms, but the pocket might eventually become inflamed, in which case the condition is called diverticulitis, characterized by pain, nausea, vomiting, low-grade fever, constipation or increased frequency of bowel movements. In severe cases, the pouch can rupture, leading to peritonitis.

- Colon Cancer is uncontrolled proliferation of cells on the inner lining of the colon. It is a common cancer and leading cause of death throughout the industrialized world.

- Leaky gut syndrome (see below)

## Leaky Gut Syndrome

At the present time, mainstream medicine does not officially recognize leaky gut syndrome, though it does recognize the existence of a leaky gut. What is the difference? A leaky gut, technically known as intestinal hyperpermeability, is exactly what it sounds like. It is the inappropriate seepage of intestinal content into the blood.

Current medical thinking regards leaky gut as the result of other pathological condition of the digestive tract. For example, leaky gut is seen as a possible consequence of irritable bowel syndrome and Crohn's disease. However, the theory of leaky gut syndrome proposes that intestinal hyperpermeability is not merely the result of other gut problems, but rather can actually *cause* them. A leaky gut is also believed to contribute to health problems beyond the gut, such as allergies, headaches, fatigue, skin rashes, joint pain, food cravings, diabetes mellites and cardiovascular disease. It has also been implicated in some autoimmune conditions, such as lupus, and rheumatoid arthritis.[6,7,8] Even psychological conditions, such as "brain fog," cognitive decline, autism, and depression might be caused by intestinal hyperpermeability.[9,10]

Some of the possible causes of leaky gut are food sensitivities, pain medication, radiation, alcohol, antibiotics, and poor diet. In other words, the usual causes are factors that we can control with lifestyle choices.

Genetic predisposition can certainly be a contributing factor in leaky gut syndrome. However, as is often the case, food acts as the trigger.[11] In fact, the so-called genetic predisposition might simply be an inability of the gut to adapt to foods and combinations of foods that are alien to our physiology. Perhaps this is why more and more medical and alternative practitioners are seeking nutritional answers to leaky gut syndrome and other gastrointestinal issues. Quite often, treatment includes some form of food combining.

# Food Combining

There is currently little hard evidence to support the idea that combining foods in specific ways will influence how well the body handles them.[12] Most of the available information is anecdotal, consisting of testimonials from patients and reports from health care providers.

What is the proper scientific response to a theory that has no hard evidence to support or refute it? The proper response is to simply withhold judgment. Furthermore, even in the absence of hard evidence, if there is a great deal of anecdotal or "soft" evidence in favor of a theory, a good scientist would acknowledge that the theory merits a closer look.

Such is the case with food combining. The evidence supporting the efficacy of food combining is virtually all anecdotal, but there is a lot of it! Some of it comes from reputable practitioners, after decades of clinical practice.[13] My personal health experience and that of my patients leads me to conclude that food combining can be very helpful, though some individuals seem to benefit from it more than others.

Will food combining help you? I cannot say for sure. However, in general, individuals with a delicate digestive system are more likely to benefit from observing the principles of food combining, compared to those who seemingly have a furnace for a stomach.

## Why does food-combining work?

The commonly accepted theory to explain why food combining works has to do with different transit times and pH requirements for the digestion of carbohydrates, fats, and protein. Whether or not this explanation is accurate and complete, the point is that good nutrition is still about relationship. In other words, the manner in which the body handles a given nutrient is influenced by the presence of other nutrients. With regard to digestion, the manner in which the body handles the carbohydrates, fats, and protein is influenced by the proportion of the three in a given meal.

We might also get a clue as to why food combining works by considering the diets of our pre-agricultural ancestors. They ate minimally processed whole foods; and typically ate one food at a time, with little or no mixing.

A given whole food typically provides the bulk of calories from either fats or carbohydrates − If one is high the other is low. In other words, *Mother Nature does not provide us with foods that have both high levels of fats and high levels of carbohydrates.*

Since our ancestors living in the wild typically ate one food at a time, they were unlikely to eat high levels of fats and carbohydrates in the same meal. The same applies to our pre-human primate ancestors — they ate that way for tens of millions of years! This eating style changed with the invention of agriculture, cooking, and food storage. Since then, the mixing of high-carb and high-fat foods into elaborate combinations have become increasingly common − and so have digestive issues.

Based on our ancestry, the ultimate form of food combining is to not combine foods at all − just eat one food at a time. However, since this is not practical for most modern humans, we can do the next best thing − we can simplify our meals. We can also *combine foods so that the proportion of fat, protein and carbohydrates resembles that of one whole food, eaten by itself.* This is precisely what food combining principles accomplish. In fact, this is what virtually every major dietary system does to optimize digestion, regulate blood sugar, and facilitate weight loss.

| |
|---|
| All well-established diets essentially practice their own version of food combining. |

66

In general, foods with higher levels of protein and fat require more time in the stomach, compared to high-carbohydrate foods. Likewise, starchy foods require more digestion than sugary foods. If we mix these different foods in substantial amounts the one that normally has a shorter transit time will be delayed, and thus become decomposed by microbes — some of which produce gas. We can avoid this by doing the following:

---

**Food Combining in a Nutshell**
- Avoid mixing large amounts of high carbohydrate foods with large amounts of high protein/fat foods.
- Avoid mixing large amounts of starchy foods with large amounts of sugary foods.

---

Here are some examples:
- If you're having a steak or other meats, go easy on the potatoes and bread.
- If you're eating potatoes, go easy on sour cream or butter.
- If you wish to eat a large serving of any sweet fruit, keep it away from the steak, potatoes, or bread.
- If you have just eaten large amounts of bread, pasta, rice, or meat, do not follow it with large amounts of a sweet dessert.

The above food combining principles may be used by anyone who wishes to optimize digestion and avoid unwanted weight gain and blood sugar issues. They can also be incorporated into the specific gut-healing diets described below.

# Gut Healing Diets

Individuals who have any of the of major illnesses of the digestive system, from hemorrhoids to cancer, can benefit dietary support. As mentioned above, all well-established diets essentially practice their own version of food combining. All of them are either carb-based (low-fat) or fat-based (low-carb). This might explain why virtually all of them, done properly, can achieve positive results, even though they might be radically different from each other. In addition, a given diet can be further modified to address specific gastro-intestinal problems. In other words, the gut healing diet may be either fat-based or carb-based.

**Fat-based Plan**

The fat-based plan that is currently popular for gut issues is the GAPS Diet.[14] The name, however, is unimportant; names come and go; diets emerge and fall out of fashion regularly. What is important is that we understand the principles on which a given diet is based. In this case, the GAPS Diet brings together a number of useful strategies for cleansing and healing the GI tract. This plan is fairly elaborate, having as many as six distinct phases. However, the essential elements are as follows:

- Eliminate starchy foods – grains, potatoes, winter squash.
- Use fruit in moderation.
- Eat generous amounts of low-starch vegetables.
- Get most of your daily calories from high-quality fat-based foods – pasture raised meats, wild caught fish, free range eggs, raw cheese, and butter, raw and perhaps sprouted nuts and seeds, avocados, coconut, coconut oil, olives, and olive oil.
- Use high quality fermented foods – sauerkraut and other cultured vegetables, yogurt, kefir, and natto.
- Use bone broth.[15] However, care should be taken to use bones from clean, pasture-raised animals, because bones store toxic metals such as lead which can accumulate in the broth.[16]
- This plan can be adjusted to suit the individual's specific gut issues. For example, if yeast overgrowth is present, you might choose to give special attention to high quality fermented foods and perhaps supplemental probiotics. If leaky gut is present, you might decide to use the amino acid L. glutamine to help restore the integrity of the inner lining of the gut.[17] If irritable bowel syndrome is present, you might consider getting tested for food allergies, so as to avoid allergenic foods as much as possible.

**Carb-based Plan**

The carb-based plan for restoring GI health can utilizes most of the strategies used by the GAPS Diet, described above. You can use most or all of the same high-quality foods – but in different proportions. The main difference is that you would reduce the fat and get the bulk of daily calories from carbohydrates – though grains are still kept to modest proportions and glutinous grains are best avoided altogether. The rest of the guidelines below are adapted from Dr. Joel Fuhrman's Eat to Live Diet, also called the Nutritarian Diet.[18]

- Three or more servings of fresh fruit per day.
- At least one pound of cooked low-starch vegetables.
- At least one pound of raw low-starch vegetables per day, including cultured vegetables.
- About one cup of cooked legumes.
- About one cup of starchy vegetables or non-glutinous grains or pseudo grains, such as brown rice, oats, or buckwheat. In general, favor starchy vegetables over grains.
- Since fatty foods are used modestly, make them count! Use nuts and seeds that provide higher levels of omega 3 oils, such as flax seeds, chia seeds and walnuts. Use the highest quality – raw, organic, and preferably soaked and sprouted.
- If you use meat or fish, do so in small amounts and get the highest quality. Bone broth is still an option. Include organ meats when possible. Prepare these foods as a hearty stew – with lots of vegetables.
- If you use dairy, favor the high-quality fermented kind – yogurt, kefir, or raw cheese – in modest proportions.
- If leaky gut or yeast are present, use fermented foods and perhaps supplemental probiotics, and L-glutamine. If IBD is present, get tested for food allergies, so as to avoid the involved foods.

## Which is Better?

Fat-based or carb-based? Some individuals seem to do okay either way, while others do better with one instead of the other. The good news is that the essential features that promote GI health are present in both dietary systems.

Either plan tends to work better with the inclusion of fermented foods and probiotics. These products inhibit growth of putrefactive bacteria – which might otherwise thrive on the higher levels of fat and protein found in fat-based diets, such as the GAPS Diet. The same fermented foods and probiotics also discourage the growth of yeast – which might otherwise thrive on the higher levels of carbohydrates found in carb-based diets.

Either plan can be followed as a temporary therapeutic diet, as described in Chapter 4, after which the person may transition to an appropriate long-term maintenance diet. This is where the guidance of a knowledgeable health professional can be beneficial.

# Tips for Digestive Health

- **Ample water**. A common cause of constipation is dehydration.
- **Lemon juice** (½-1 lemon) in warm water every morning. This will encourage digestion and promote liver cleansing.
- **Plant fiber.** Get enough to allow for at least one bowel movement per day. The best sources are raw fruits and vegetables.
- **Dark green leafy vegetables**, especially dandelion and kale provide extra liver support.
- **Eat when you're hungry.** And stop when you are full! A common contributor to indigestion is eating for reasons other than true hunger. We tend to eat out of habit, nervousness, or because we are at a social gathering. In addition, we frequently eat pre-set portions and feel obligated to "clean the plate" rather than eating the amount the body calls for.
- **Peppermint tea** makes for a pleasant beverage that promotes good digestion. Peppermint tea is readily available in health food stores in tea bags or in bulk.
- **Fennel and ginger tea**. Make a tea of fennel seeds and fresh ginger. Cut up one ounce of fresh ginger and place in a one-quart mason glass with 3 tablespoons of fennel seeds. Fill the jar with very hot (almost boiling) water and let steep for at least half an hour. Peppermint may also be added.
- **Probiotics and fermented foods**. Sauerkraut, yogurt, and probiotic supplements promote a healthy population of intestinal microorganisms. This is especially important if you are taking antimicrobial agents, such as antibiotics.
- **Aloe Vera** is cleaning and healing for the GI tract. Its anti-inflammatory and regenerative properties can be beneficial for inflammatory or degenerative conditions of the gut. It has antimicrobial properties that can help eliminate intestinal pathogens, while sparing beneficial bacteria![19] It supports the immune system and might therefore be helpful for individuals with Crone's disease, colitis, or cancer. Its powerful regenerative properties can help heal damage due to hemorrhoids, ulcers, leaky gut, and other degenerative conditions.

# Chapter 7
# Breathing Freely

The Key to Respiratory Health
The Respiratory Tree
Respiratory Cures

Prior to the discovery of penicillin by Alexander Fleming in 1928, respiratory infections such as pneumonia and tuberculosis were often fatal. In fact, respiratory infections were a major cause of death in those days. Hospitals and sanitariums specializing in tuberculosis were common in Europe and the Americas until the 1930s.

Today, death from respiratory infections is far less common due to indoor plumbing, better sanitation, and easy access to strong antibiotics. Nonetheless, upper, and lower respiratory infections are still quite common, as are non-infectious respiratory conditions such as asthma, bronchitis, allergies, and cancer. In fact, we might say that respiratory issues are as common as digestive issues — which apparently is not a mere coincidence. In one sense, the key to respiratory health is digestive health.

## The Key to Respiratory Health

The connection between gut-health and respiratory health seems logical when we remember that a hefty chunk of our immunity comes from a thriving population of intestinal bacteria. However, the connection runs deeper than that.

Congestion in the digestive system seems to trigger congestion in the air passages. The reason becomes clear when we remember that the lungs do more than just take in oxygen and expel carbon dioxide. The respiratory system also serves as a means for removing waste products that the body is unable to adequately expel through other portals of elimination. As an example, the day after heavy alcohol consumption, the breath is likely to smell like alcohol.

More commonly, when the digestive tract and liver become overburdened with waste products from a poorly functioning digestive system, the respiratory system is pressed into service. It becomes a dumping ground for all manner of toxic substances and allergens which are generated by putrefactive bacteria, yeast, and larger parasites in the gut. The presence of leaky gut, described in the previous chapter, can aggravate the problem.

The result is that the respiratory system becomes more vulnerable to infectious and non-infectious conditions. To complicate matters, when an individual takes antibiotics to get rid of a respiratory infection, the beneficial bacteria in the gut are decimated, which further compromises the immune system. For example, some clinicians have reported that children with strep throat who were treated with antibiotics recovered faster but seemed more likely to have future recurrence of the condition. One explanation given for this observation was that the antibiotics killed the beneficial bacteria in the throat.[1]

| The key to respiratory health is digestive health. |
|---|

Research is now validating the ancient principle of promoting respiratory health through digestive health.[2] Beyond that, we can also use foods, herbs, and supplements to directly address respiratory problems. To understand how we can best use such products, let us first the basic anatomy and physiology of the respiratory system.

## The Respiratory Tree

The respiratory system is essentially a series of air passages that resemble an upside-down tree. The trunk of the tree consists of the nasal cavity, throat, larynx (voice box), and trachea (windpipe).

In the upper chest, the trachea branches into two bronchi, each of which enters one lung and branches again into a series of smaller air passages. The terminal branches (the twigs of the tree) are studded with numerous microscopic air-filled domes. To the early anatomists examining the microscopic architecture of the lungs, these domes resembled grapes and were therefore named "alveoli," which is the Latin word for "grapes."

If we imagine that the respiratory tree is more like a grapevine, the alveoli do, indeed, look like thick clusters of grapes. There are approximately 300 million of these grapes in each lung.

Alveoli are the business end of the respiratory system. They provide a hugely important interface between the blood and air passages, allowing oxygen to enter the blood, while carbon dioxide and other waste products leave the blood.

Alveoli within lungs

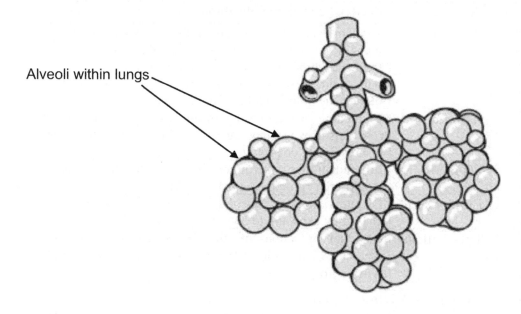

## What About Sinuses?

Individuals suffering from sinus problems — which include a rather large percentage of humans — might be wondering where sinuses fit into the respiratory tree (or grapevine), described above. Sinuses are technically not part of the respiratory tree; they are distinct air-filled chambers or caves within the bones of the forehead and cheeks. This is why we might feel pressure in the forehead or cheeks when the sinuses are inflamed by an infection or air-born allergens.

The sinuses in the forehead and face do have small openings that drain into the nasal cavity, but the air that we breathe doesn't have to actually pass through them. This is why we can still breathe freely even when we have "stuffy" sinuses. In contrast, when the nose is stuffy, we would suffocate if we didn't have a secondary passage for air – the mouth.

| Common Respiratory Ailments | |
|---|---|
| Name | Description |
| Common Cold | Viral infection of the nasal cavity, characterized by sneezing, runny nose, nasal congestion, and cough. |
| Influenza (flu) | Viral infection characterized by fever, chills, headaches, and muscular ache. |
| Strep throat | Bacterial infection of the throat. |
| Pneumonia | Viral or bacterial infection of the air passages of the lungs. Prior to the use of antibiotics, this condition was frequently fatal, because the smaller air passages can fill with fluid, thus preventing oxygen from reaching the blood. The individual literally drowns. |
| Asthma | Tightening of the muscles of air passages in the lungs, resulting in wheezing, tightness of the chest, shortness of breath, and coughing. |
| Bronchitis | Inflammation of the inner lining of the air passages resulting in chronic cough and shortness of breath. |
| Emphysema | Disintegration of alveoli. The condition is usually caused by exposure to cigarette smoke. |
| Tuberculosis | Bacterial infection of the lungs characterized by coughing with blood-tinged sputum, fever, and weight loss. |

**Ending the Vicious Cycle**

The inability to exercise could prevent full recovery from a chronic respiratory condition. Consequently, the person gets caught in a vicious cycle wherein the respiratory ailment restricts exercise which in turn further compromises respiratory health and eventually takes a toll on the body as a whole.

One of the benefits of using good nutrition for respiratory health is that the individual might get enough relief to allow regular exercise which then allows for even deeper cleansing and healing of the respiratory passages. In this manner, the vicious cycle of degeneration is transformed into a positive-feedback cycle of increasing health. This is yet another example of how good nutrition and exercise can work synergistically; each enhancing the other; and both working together to produce results that are greater than the mere sum of the two.

# Respiratory Relief

- **Grapes** are good for the lungs in general, especially asthma and bronchitis.[3] Resveratrol in grapes has been shown to reduce inflammation and viral replication in lower respiratory infections in children.[4]
- **Figs, oranges, freshly squeezed orange juice, fresh pineapple, lemon, lemon juice, lemon peel, cilantro,** and **grapes** may be helpful in cleansing and decongesting the upper and lower respiratory passages.
- **Garlic** is a powerful detoxifier and antimicrobial agent. Fresh and raw garlic is stronger than cooked, but the latter is also helpful when used as a condiment or taken in capsules.
- **Ginger** may be used in capsules or as a tea. The most potent form is freshly squeezed ginger juice diluted with water or other juices. Fresh ginger may also be blended with cilantro, lemon, and warm water, making a potent tonic for the respiratory and digestive systems. Garlic may also be added.
- **Noni juice** can be beneficial as a respiratory tonic. Among its virtues, it is reputed to have antimicrobial properties.
- **Aloe vera** can be helpful for inflammatory conditions of the respiratory system, such as infections, allergic reactions, and other irritants.
- **For asthma**, common remedies include grapes, grape juice, cranberry juice, lemon juice, mint, noni juice, and ginger. Since asthma is often associated with allergies, modulating of the immune system as described in chapter 13 can also be very helpful.
- **For sinus support**, N-acetyl cysteine may be helpful. My patients who have taken it have reported a purging of the sinuses, followed by a feeling of relief from stuffiness. According to one theory, chronic sinus issues involve mucus becoming dry and gummy, perhaps exacerbated by the drying effect of antihistamines — which are often taken for sinus issues. Eventually, mucus gets caked on the walls of the sinuses, providing a haven for bacteria. N-acetyl cysteine seems to flush out the mucus along with bacteria. Some versions of this product combine N-acetyl cysteine with certain beneficial bacteria that support the immune system.

# Chapter 8
# Skin & Hair

Our Third Kidney
Cleansing and Nourishing the Skin
Fat-based Diet or Carb-based Diet

As with the rest of the body, our skin, hair, and nails suffer when they are deprived of nutrients and overburdened with toxicity. The difference is that skin, hair and nails are external and therefore visible.

A healthy exterior is not just an end in itself. Degenerative changes in the skin, hair, and nails are visible indicators of internal problems which might otherwise be invisible — though far more serious in terms of their effects on overall health and longevity. Acne, psoriasis, nail fungus, athletes foot, jock itch, ringworm, wrinkling of skin, loss of skin pigmentation, graying of hair, warts, skin cancer, dermatitis, eczema, sunburn, age spots and other forms of sun damage, are all very visible. They can also be prevented and often reversed with good nutrition. And, in so doing, we often help correct the associated internal conditions which cause skin problem.

To understand the above-mentioned skin issues, including how to improve them with good nutrition, let us first take a look at the structure and function of skin. The skin is not just a lifeless barrier. It is alive, very complex, and serves a number of vital functions. Most notably, the skin has been called the "third kidney."

## Our Third Kidney

Sweat, like urine, is a mixture of chemicals consisting of waste products. In fact, sweat is chemically similar to urine. The process of perspiration, whether visible or invisible, is an important way of cleansing the body. The average person produces about one quart of sweat per day, which is comparable to the volume of urine produced by each kidney. In addition, during vigorous exercise, the skin might produce the same amount of sweat in just one hour.

The skin has also been called the "third lung" because it can absorb oxygen directly from the atmosphere, though this is not as critically important as once believed.[1] The skin, like the rest of the body, receives oxygen from the lungs, but also receives it from the surrounding air. The point is that we are in no danger of suffocating if we temporarily lose the ability to absorb oxygen directly through the skin. If the oxygen absorbed through the skin was indeed critically important to meet the body's oxygen requirements, scuba divers would not be able to survive very long underwater — with their skin completely covered in a tight-fitting rubber suite. Nonetheless, for optimal health, we should let the skin "breathe." In addition to the direct benefit to the skin, the bodys's ability to *sense* oxygen through the skin seems to be an important way in which the body regulates its levels of nitric oxide.[2]

## Know Thy Skin

The skin has two main layers. The outer layer is called the epidermis, which consists of closely packed cells, rich in a tough protein called keratin. The deeper layer is called the dermis which consists of loosely scattered cells, surrounded by a dense network of collagen threads, blood vessels, nerves, sweat glands, oil glands, and hair roots.

Hair and nails are essentially made of dead epidermal cells which are especially rich in keratin. The cells of the epidermis reproduce rapidly and are eventually worn off at the surface. The entire epidermis is replaced in about 90 days. The reason why tattoos are permanent is that the dye is injected down into the dermis, which is much more stable than the epidermis.

### Cross Section of Skin

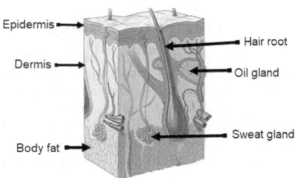

Once we understand the basic construction of the skin, common skin problems start to make sense so we can get a clue as to how to correct them. For example:

- Pimples are due to clogged and infected oil glands.
- Skin cancer, warts, and psoriasis are examples of abhorrent skin growth due to abnormally rapid division of epidermal cells. Skin cancer has been attributed to DNA damage from ultraviolet rays.
- Sunburn, dermatitis, eczema, and other skin rashes are just inflammation, made possible by the abundant blood vessels in the dermis.
- Wrinkling, loss of elasticity, and leathery appearance of skin are largely due to free radical damage to the collagen in the dermis.
- Scars are due to damaged collagen in the dermis that does not regenerate properly.

## Cleansing and Nourishing the Skin

### Aloe Vera

Aloe Vera has been used for thousands of years for multiple health issues, including psoriasis, skin ulcers, sun-burn, dandruff, and skin rashes. Its benefits for the skin are so obvious and often dramatic that we might forget that it has equally beneficial effects for the rest of the body. Studies show that aloe vera is anti-inflammatory, antibacterial, and antimicrobial. It also seems to jump-start tissue regeneration, which might explain why it reportedly promotes healthy skin, hair, and nails. It can benefit the skin when used topically or internally.

### Colorful fruits and Vegetables

Sun damage to skin is essentially the same as the damage done by other forms of radiation. How *does* radiation damage tissue? It damages tissue by triggering production of free radicals in the body. Free radical damage can trigger skin cancer in the already rapidly dividing cells of the epidermis. The same free radicals can also age the skin by causing damage to the collagen in the dermis. This is why antioxidants are important for the long-term health and youthfulness of skin. Our best source of antioxidants are colorful fruits and vegetables.

## Coconut and Coconut Oil

Ingesting whole coconut and coconut oil, as well as applying the oil topically, have been used for a number of skin problems, including dry scaly skin, dermatitis, eczema and psoriasis. It seems to benefit the skin in at least three ways:

- It contains polyphenols, which have strong antioxidant properties.
- The medium chain triglycerides in coconut oil have antibacterial and antifungal properties.
- The medium-chain triglycerides also have an affinity for keratin, which might partially explain why coconut oil can help promote hair growth and skin regeneration.[3]

As a point of caution, hair *loss* has also been reported with the application of coconut oil to the scalp. In addition, regarding its internal use, remember that coconut oil is not a whole food. As with other extracted oils, it is a concentrated form of fat-calories. If used mindlessly, the calories will add up fast. Therefore, use it conservatively. Experienced users of coconut oil have learned that a little is great, but a lot is not. I would suggest that for internal use, you replace some of the coconut oil with whole coconut when possible. Whole coconut is more nutritionally balanced and less likely to be overconsumed. Appendix E gives a more detailed description of coconut oil.

## Omega 3 Oils

Omega 3 oils, used topically and internally, help moisturize skin and reduce the severity of rashes from dermatitis and eczema. Research also indicates that omega 3 oils can reduce acne.[4] There is also evidence suggesting that omega 3 supplementation could help prevent and treat certain types of skin cancer.[5] As with coconut oil, omega 3 supplements are best when used conservatively and judiciously; take the amount needed to achieve the desired results and avoid excess. In addition to being subject to the same limitations as other oils (very concentrated fat-calories), omega 3 oils also happen to be highly sensitive to free radical damage.

## Fat Soluble Vitamins

Vitamins A, D and E help moisturize, protect, and heal the skin. All three can be taken internally in supplement form. They are also available as topical creams to help various skin conditions, including dry skin, psoriasis, and various forms of skin rashes, including diaper rash.

## Silicon

This mineral is much loved by the skin. It is needed to make collagen in the dermis. It is also believed to contribute to healthy hair and nails by transporting other essential minerals to the skin.

Not surprisingly, deficiencies can lead to thinning hair, brittle nails and aging of skin. Silicon is found abundantly in apples, oranges, lettuce, cucumbers, tomatoes, cabbage, onions, whole grains, and almonds. In addition, the herb horse-tail may be taken in supplement form or as a tea to provide the body with extra silicon. Silicon is frequently included in skin care products.

## Sulfur

This is another mineral that is loved by skin. The keratin making up skin, hair, and nails is rich in sulfur. That is why burning hair smells like rotten eggs.

We usually get sulfur as part of two amino acids called cysteine and methionine. It is also found in thiamine (vitamin B1) and biotin, both very good for the skin. Onions, garlic, broccoli, cauliflower, kale, cabbage, and Brussels sprouts are rich in sulfur-containing phytonutrients.

# Dry Skin Brushing

Exfoliation is the process of removing dead cells which have piled up on the surface of the skin. The accumulation of dead cells contributes to a dull, dry, or rough appearance. In addition, the debris can contribute to clogging of pores and oil glands, leading to blemishes.

Deep exfoliation may occasionally be done with acids applied by an esthetician. However, a gentler version can also be done at home with something that mildly abrasive, such as a dry towel, sponge, or loofa. Either way, exfoliated skin looks and functions better. It can receive nourishment from the blood more easily, as well as excrete more freely and perhaps absorb oxygen from the air more readily.

The dry-brush method also has a massaging action which stimulates sweat glands, oil glands, hair follicles, and directly benefits circulation of blood and lymph in the dermis. In addition, the dry-brush method is easier, less expensive, and safer than chemical exfoliation, which means that it can be done on a regular basis and thus provide the added benefits of long-term use — deeper cleansing and healing of the skin and the rest of the body. With regular dry skin brushing, the nutritional measures described below will be more available to the skin.

## Fat-based Diet or Carb-based Diet?

As described in Chapter 2, the presence of both large amounts of fats and carbohydrates in the same diet, and especially in the same meal, increase the likelihood of overeating, indigestion, and blood sugar issues, all of which can eventually contribute to skin problems. The simple solution is to eat either a carb-based (low-fat) or fat-based (low-carb) diet. Your skin will let you know which one it prefers.

If you tend to get athlete's foot, jock-itch, nail fungus and dry skin, you might do better with a fat-base diet, which means that you get the bulk of your calories from fats, while limiting your carbs. On the other hand, if you tend to get pimples, oily skin, or oily hair, and body odor, you would probably do well with a carb-based diet, which means that you would get the bulk of your calories from carbohydrates, while limiting your fats.

As a point of caution, if you choose the carb-based (low-fat) approach, make sure the diet is not *too* low in fat. Have enough high-quality fats in your diet, especially omega 3, to keep the skin moisturized and happy. In other words, with a carb-based diet, be modest with fats, but make them count!

If you don't have a clear sense of which dietary direction to take, the simple solution is to try one or the other and pay attention to the results. The diet which produces the most benefit to your skin, hair, and nails will probably also produce the most benefit to the rest of your body as well.

Either way, favor whole foods, including a goodly amount of fresh produce. In particular, favor fruits and vegetables that are rich in silicon, sulfur, and antioxidants, as described above.

# Chapter 9
# Food & Stress

What is Stress?
Stress Begets More Stress
Food as a Stress Inducer
Integrated Stress Reduction Program
Food as a Stress Reducer

The connection between stress and food runs deep, with the arrow of influence pointing in both directions. In other words, stress influences how we eat; and how we eat can influence how well the body handles various stressors.

Until recently, stress received little medical attention because it did not seem to be associated with any of the major diagnosable illnesses. Individuals who went to a medical doctor complaining of being "tense" or unable to sleep properly were just told to get some rest or take a drug — or both. The stressed-out patient who also complained of physical pain which had no apparent cause, was often dismissed as neurotic. All this is changing.

There is now general agreement among health professionals that stress merits close attention. Thus far, the data point to one stark conclusion: stress kills.

Stress has been associated with virtually all major degenerative diseases of civilization.[1] Stress has been linked with cardiovascular disease, which is still the leading cause of death in industrialized nations. It is also linked to cancer, the second leading cause of death. Stress-reduction is being incorporated into the day-to-day practice of various health care providers, including medical doctors, chiropractors, osteopaths, naturopaths, and massage therapists.

The first step in effectively reducing and reversing the harmful effects of stress is to gain a clear understanding as to what it really is and how it impacts our physiology.

# What is Stress?

In the language of physiology, stress is anything that challenges the body's ability to maintain itself in a healthy state. More specifically, stress is any *change* in the inner or outer environment that challenges the body's ability to maintain equilibrium with regard to blood pressure, blood sugar, cholesterol levels, hormone levels, body temperature, pH, digestion, immune function, etc.

Using the above definition, stress does not necessarily have to be harmful. In fact, the right kind and right amount of stress is considered necessary for maintaining health. Therefore, researchers make a distinction between *eustress* (good stress) and *distress* (bad stress). For example, stress in the form of moderate exercise is considered eustress because it is essential for maintaining strong bones and muscles, as well as helping to maintain clean and healthy arteries, strong immune system, proper blood pressure, blood sugar levels, cholesterol levels, digestion, respiration, mental clarity, and emotional serenity.

However, when stress is excessive or of the wrong kind, we may call it *distress* because it can overtax and eventually overpower the body's ability to maintain inner equilibrium. The result? The body undergoes a number of unhealthy physiological changes. The technical term for these changes is General Adaptation Syndrome (GAS).

## Do You Have GAS?

The most obvious short-term effects of stress are fatigue, mood swings, depression, digestive disturbance, asthmatic attack, unrestful sleep, and craving sweets. The long-term effects may include a depressed immune system, allergies, fibromyalgia, cardiovascular disease, cancer, diabetes mellitus, and death of brain cells.

When the body goes into general adaptation syndrome, it becomes depleted of energy and other resources. This and other changes reduce the body's ability to repair and regenerate, as well as creating internal conditions that favor the onset of many degenerative conditions. Bottom line, a stressed-out body ages faster and is more vulnerable to illness.[2]

## The Physiology of Stress

The original work on stress was done by Hans Selye MD.[3] As a medical student in 1926, he found that the body shows the same basic reactions to stress, regardless of the source — infection, chemical toxicity, or psychological disturbances. Here are some physiological effects of stress:

- Raises blood pressure
- Thickens the blood
- Raises blood sugar
- Raises platelet count – higher risk of clot formation
- Raises serum cholesterol levels
- Accelerates dying of brain cells
- Produces low-grade inflammation which, in turn, leads to a variety of degenerative diseases.

Dr. Selye also stated that the body's response to stress occurs in three phases:

- **Phase 1: Alarm Phase**. The body reacts to stress with an outpouring of stress hormones from the adrenal glands. The main stress hormones are adrenalin and cortisol. These two hormones mobilize the body's energy to adapt to the stressful situation. Most individuals associate the adrenal glands with heavy exercise or heightened emotions, both of which can produce the so-called adrenalin rush. Less obvious but equally significant, the same adrenal alarm can be activated by infections, drugs, and certain foods. If the stressful event is brief, the body quickly recovers. If the stress continues, the body eventually moves into phase two.

- **Phase 2: Resistance Phase**. The body tries to adapt to the ongoing stress by breaking down tissues to mobilize needed nutrients. In this phase, the individual might feel fine and may actually feel great — because stress hormones inhibit pain and inflammation, while perhaps giving the person an energetic lift or "buzz." However, phase 2 is like living on credit cards. If the person starts out with good credit, in the form of robust health and a substantial bank-account of nutrient reserves, phase 2 can go on for a long time. However, the body is gradually depleted and eventually moves into phase 3.

- **Phase 3: Exhaustion Phase**. This phase is often called "adrenal exhaustion." The minor aches and pains, occasional insomnia, and moodiness progress into more serious conditions.

Injuries are more likely to happen and healing occurs more slowly. Years of fluctuating blood sugar becomes diabetes mellitus. The gradual stripping away of calcium from the bones shows up as osteoporosis and fractures. The accelerated killing of brain cells due to chronically high cortisol levels eventually shows up as senile dementia. The disruption of the immune system shows up as a greater propensity for respiratory infections and allergies. The stress-induced thickening of blood and high blood pressure, which had been silently irritating the kidneys and clogging of the arteries over a period of years, can eventually show up as kidney failure or heart disease.

**Accumulating Stress**

Since all stressors effect the body in essentially the same way, they can easily have a cumulative effect. In other words, one stressor acting alone might be handled with ease and grace, but many low-grade stressors, acting together or sequentially, can overpower the body's capacity for self-regulation just as easily as one very large and obvious stressor. For example, a person might be able to cope with low-grade stress at work, but when other stressors show up, such as a rapid change in the weather or loss of a loved one, the body is no longer able to cope.

The specific health problems that emerge can vary from person to person, but the general pattern may be summarized as follows: tissues become dehydrated, the vital organs and glands gradually shrink and the body ages faster.

# Stress Begets More Stress

When the body goes deeply enough into GAS, a vicious cycle is set up wherein the condition becomes self-perpetuating. For example, too much stress during the day prevents the body from resting at night. This is due to stress hormones remaining high, even after going to bed. The next day, the person may have low energy and therefore takes a stimulant, such as coffee, which stresses the body even more and perpetuates the cycle.

The morning coffee, without which many individuals would find it difficult to start the day, is followed by a coffee break a few hours later, and maybe a few more cups in the afternoon, along with the extra caffeine from soft drinks and chocolate candy.

In one sense, when the body goes deeply enough into GAS, it "forgets" how to properly restore itself. For example, in addition to general sleeplessness, the individual has a harder time reaching deep dreamless sleep, during which the pituitary gland normally sends out a surge of growth hormone (GH) that promotes regeneration. The individual cannot relax and is trapped in a self-perpetuating loop in which the body literally breaks itself down at an ever-increasing rate.

## Endless Internal War

To complete our understanding of how chronic stress impacts the body, let us consider the autonomic nervous system. This is the part of the nervous system which regulates our internal organs and glands. The autonomic system is said to have two parts or divisions: the sympathetic and parasympathetic divisions.

The parasympathetic division allows the body to rest and regenerate. For example, it slows the heart, slows breathing and promotes digestion. In contrast, the sympathetic division promotes activities that expend energy. For example, sympathetic stimulation tends to increase heart rate, increases the rate and depth of respiration, and inhibits digestion.

Massive dominance of the sympathetic division is called the fight-or-flight response, which allows the body to cope with life-threatening situations. When the body is in a state of GAS, it is essentially stuck in chronic, low-grade fight-or-flight.[4] The body is perpetually in battle-mode; a state of hyper-vigilance which disrupts our restorative functions.

As the condition progresses and symptoms worsen, the individual might go from one desperate measure to another, trying to put out little fires by doing things that start new fires — such as taking drugs that eventually necessitate even more drugs.

The central issue here is that the body perceives itself as being under attack but is unable to successfully defeat the "enemy" because the attack is coming from within. Indeed, the body is being attacked by the very systems which are supposed to defend and protect it. For example, the immune system attacks the body's own tissue (autoimmune conditions) while the endocrine system secretes hormones that inhibit regeneration, while adding to the general state of hypervigilance. The body does not realize that the only way to win this battle is to just stop fighting.

# Food as a Stress Inducer

Stress, especially emotional stress, often drives us to seek comfort in the form of food. The usual comfort foods tend to require a lot of digestion and clean-up — which stress the body even more. This is a prime example of stress begetting more stress. Here are some of the common food sources of stress:

- Overconsumption of calories, especially in the form of refined and highly processed foods, can ring the adrenal alarm, and release stress hormones.[5]

- The presence of additives and irritants in food will ring the adrenal alarm even louder.

- Mineral imbalance is another subtle but powerful way in which we drive the body toward GAS. The typical diet in industrialized regions is rich in sodium, which tends stimulate nerves, induce muscle tension, and raise blood pressure. The same diet tends to be deficient in potassium, magnesium, and perhaps calcium, all of which promote relaxation.

- Coffee seems to have some real benefits, at least for some individuals, as described in Appendix A. However, it can become yet another way of overstimulating the adrenal glands and therefore pushing the body further into GAS. As described in Chapter 4, any substance which has the potential to change our physiology for the better, can also change it for the worse, if not used with care. Caffeine is an irritant, and that is how it stimulates the adrenal glands. Caffeine is the most widely used drug in the world.[6]

- Eating a lot of meat tends to raise the levels of stress hormones. Red meat raises the level of uric acid which affects the body in a manner similar to caffeine — it stimulates the release of cortisol.[7]

- Soft drinks are corrosive to the body, triggering a number of problems such as blood sugar issues, mood swings, tooth decay and osteoporosis. Colas also represent yet another source of artificial caffeine. However, here again, the problem with soft drinks is the large amount that many people consume. Limiting consumption is certainly helpful but doing so might be tricky because, whether or not it is intentional, these products are formulated in a way that makes them rather addictive.

- MSG (monosodium glutamate) is a flavor enhancer developed in the early 20th century. It was originally used only in Asian restaurants but is now used widely in fast-food restaurants and packaged food. According to neurosurgeon and author Russell Blaylock MD, MSG is an excitotoxin; it kills brain cells by over-exciting them. He also points out that it would be meaningless to speak of safe levels of MSG, because the amounts that are needed to enhance the flavor of food are the same amounts that kill brain cells.[8]

> By minimizing exposure to stressors that we can regulate, such as food, we empower the body to neutralize the effects of the remaining stressors.

## Integrated Stress Reduction Program

Just as stress-inducing agents tend have a cumulative effect, so do stress-reducing activities. Here are several ways of de-stressing the body and mind.

- **Rest**. The body must have quiet time in order to recover its energy and regenerate. This is difficult with a stressed individual because body is in a state of hypervigilance wherein it has a hard time relaxing. This is where the suggestions below can be very helpful.

- **Exercise** is one the simplest and most effective ways of helping the body remember how to rest. It also promotes good circulation, digestion, strong bones, and muscles, normalizing blood pressure and balancing blood sugar and cholesterol. Exercise facilitates deep, restful sleep, which further promotes regeneration. Many of these benefits may be attributed to elevated nitric oxide levels which occur with regular exercise. The trick to succeeding with exercise is to start slow and go easy. Increase your time and intensity at a gradual rate, to avoid getting discouraged or injured.

- **Massage Therapy** is one of the most potent therapeutic tools to get the body out of General Adaptation Syndrome. One reason that massage is so effective is that the session typically lasts an hour, during which the person is lying still while soothing music is playing in the background. Therefore, the body can reach deeper levels of relaxation compared to other therapies that are applied for a shorter time and in a less restful environment. For optimal results, a series of massage treatments (10-12), about one per week are recommended.

- **Give Yourself 90 Days**. Any health-promoting activity done consistently for three months is likely to make a significant change. In this case, the program might include regular exercise, rest, massage, and good nutrition. Together, they help the body greatly reduce the short-term and long-term effects of stress, while also promoting health and longevity in other ways.

- **Good Nutrition**. Just as food can be a major stressor, it can also be a powerful stress reducer, as described below.

# Food as a Stress Reducer

The body responds to different stressors in pretty much the same way, which means that all stressors tend to have a cumulative effect. Therefore, by minimizing exposure to stressors that we can regulate, such as food, we empower the body to neutralize the effects of remaining stressors. This is how we can avoid drifting ever deeper into the vicious cycle of stress begetting more stress. By simply selecting the cleanest and most nutritious foods possible, we empower the body to neutralize the effects of air pollution, water pollution, computer screens, cell phones, and the various forms of mental and emotional stress that we encounter daily.

In addition to the general guidelines for healthy eating described in Chapter 4, we can make specific adjustments to give the body the added resources it needs to effectively move though stressful periods. The nutrients which are depleted most readily by stress are vitamin C, B vitamins, several minerals, antioxidants, amino acids, and omega 3 oils. Therefore, we would select foods that provide ample amounts of these nutrients — in the cleanest and most digestible form possible. For example:

- Cold water fish and free-range eggs are good sources of amino acids, beneficial fats, fat-soluble nutrients, and some minerals.

- Nuts, seeds, legumes, sea vegetation, buckwheat, and mushrooms are good plant sources of micronutrients, amino acids, and beneficial fats. Algae oil is a good source of omega 3 oils in the form of DHA and EPA.

- Homemade soups and stews are an excellent way of preparing the above-mentioned foods. Regarding meat, try to include organ meats and bones, because these are loaded with nutrients to help replenish a stressed out and depleted body. Also, by making soups and stews rather than baking, broiling, or frying, you can minimize loss of nutrients and production of toxic byproducts associated with high-temperature cooking.

- With animal products, it is especially important to choose the highest quality. There is a major difference between meat, eggs and dairy from factory-farmed animals compared to the same products from a local, organic farm. It is also important not to over-consume animal products, meat in particular, because that would constitute another source of stress. The good news is that the beneficial substances in animal products that might be missing or deficient in plant foods are concentrated enough to allow us to get enough of the needed nutrients even when these foods are consumed in modest amounts.

- Culinary herbs such as cumin, turmeric and oregano have health-promoting properties and reduce the need for salt.

- Make room for fresh fruits and vegetables. They are the cleanest and easiest to digest of all food groups which means the body has more energy available to neutralize the effects of stress. In addition, they are the richest source of vitamin C, most B vitamins, minerals and antioxidants which help to destress the body in a number of ways, as described below.

**The Stress-reducing Power of Fresh Produce**

Vitamin C, B vitamins, and minerals are of central importance for reducing pain and promoting relaxation. In particular, potassium, magnesium and calcium help relax muscles, alkalize the body, and soothe the nervous system. All three are depleted during stressful periods. All three are abundant in fruits and vegetables. Dark green leafy vegetables tend to be rich in calcium.

In addition to providing alkalizing minerals, fruits and vegetables provide flavonoids, some of which enhance mental clarity, emotional serenity, cheerfulness, and muscular relaxation. They do so mostly by promoting higher levels of certain neurotransmitters (such as serotonin) and hormones (such as melatonin). Flavonoids are especially abundant in fruits high in vitamin C, such as citrus, strawberries, kiwi, pineapple, papaya, and mangos. Brain benefitting flavonoids are also available in many herbs and teas such as ginkgo biloba, chamomile, St. John's wart, and passionflower. These herbs have traditionally been used to promote positive mental and emotion states.

# Chapter 10
# Pain and Inflammation

The Cause of Chronic Pain
Fibromyalgia
Dietary Stressors and Pain
Food for Pain Relief

In order to effectively address pain, we must first recognize that it has an important function. Pain is how our innate intelligence lets our educated intelligence know that something is out of balance. Therefore, the proper way to treat a painful condition is to correct the imbalance which causes the pain. On the other hand, if we merely block the perception of pain while neglecting its cause, the imbalance persists and the body continues to silently degenerate.

Granted, when pain is severe or unrelenting, it does become a problem in and of itself; it becomes yet another source of stress that contributes to degeneration. Nonetheless, the basic strategy is still the same: stop the pain as quickly as possible and do so in a way that resolves the underlying cause.

## The Cause of Chronic Pain

In many cases, the cause of chronic pain is a reduction of blood flow in a given area. Even when lack of blood flow isn't the primary cause, it can still contribute to the problem.

Why does lack of blood supply result in pain? Reduced circulation means reduced oxygen. Reduced oxygen means the cells in the area will have a harder time generating enough energy to function properly. Nerve cells often respond to lack of energy by becoming hypersensitive, eventually becoming damaged. Here are some examples of pain associated with lack of oxygen.

- **Angina pectoris** is pain on the left side of the chest, perhaps extending into the left arm. This is a common example of pain due to lack of oxygen. In this case, it signals lack of oxygen to the heart muscle.

- **Diabetic neuropathy** is pain, mainly in the extremities, associated with diabetes mellites. It is due to reduced blood flow and eventually leads to nerve damage.
- **CRPS** (Complex Regional Pain Syndrome) is inflammation and burning pain, usually in one or more of the extremities. It typically starts several months after a traumatic injury.
- **Chemotherapy** often results in pain because the drugs destroy small blood vessels, thus depriving tissues of oxygen.
- **Cholesterol-lowering drugs** can cause neuropathy by depleting coenzyme $Q_{10}$. Inadequate levels of coenzyme $Q_{10}$ prevent the local cells from generating enough energy.
- **Raynaud's syndrome** is a condition in which spasm of arteries result in reduced blood flow, usually in the fingers and less commonly the toes.
- **Osteoarthritis.** The pain and tenderness with this condition seem to be linked to circulation and oxygen.
- **Fibromyalgia.** The pain associated with this condition seem to be linked to circulation. However, this condition is more than a circulatory condition, as described below.

# Fibromyalgia

In the past, individuals exhibiting signs of fibromyalgia were often dismissed as neurotics or hypochondriacs. However, with increased awareness of the effects of stress on the body, we now know that fibromyalgia syndrome is yet another pathological condition that can develop after years of stress.[1]

Here are some of the major symptoms:
- Widespread pain and stiffness, especially in the morning
- Persistent fatigue, anxiety, and depression
- Non-refreshing sleep

Pain from fibromyalgia is associated with a certain type of tissue called fibrous connective tissue – hence the name, *fibro*myalgia. This tissue is the glue which holds together our joints, muscles, bones, and skin. Given the widespread distribution of fibrous connective tissue, we can easily see why the pain of fibromyalgia is also widespread.

## The Collagen Connection

Fibrous connective tissue is called "fibrous" because it derives its strength from countless microscopic threads made of a protein called collagen, which is by far the most abundant protein in the body. If a person suddenly became invisible except for the collagen, we would still be able to recognize the person from the intricate collagen matrix permeating the body.

The body places a high priority on maintaining the integrity of it collagenous tissues. What does this have to do with fibromyalgia? Quite simply, in fibromyalgia the body's ability to maintain integrity of its collagen matrix has been compromised.

What does the body need to make collagen? The primary requirements are protein and vitamin C. Generally, getting enough protein is not a problem. Most individuals eating the typical modern diet get lots of protein. However, that same diet also tends to be very low in vitamin C.

Furthermore, when the body is subjected to chronic stress, which is typical for individuals suffering from fibromyalgia, vitamin C is used up more quickly. Therefore, deficiency is probable and collagen production can be compromised. In addition, the same stressors that use up vitamin C and provoke other imbalances, such as hormonal issues which can also translate into a greater propensity for degeneration and pain, as described below.

## The Hormone Connection

Many symptoms of fibromyalgia may be attributed to overproduction of stress hormones such as cortisol, as described on the previous chapter. Cortisol, among its many actions, triggers collagen breakdown. The same stressful conditions that provoke higher cortisol levels are also likely to induce under-production of restorative hormones such as growth hormone (GH). Growth hormone promotes collagen production.

In addition to directly triggering collagen breakdown, high levels of cortisol also result in disturbed sleep. More specifically, individuals with fibromyalgia do not get adequate amounts of "delta" sleep – a deep dreamless sleep, during which the pituitary gland sends out its biggest surge of growth hormone, thus allowing the body to carry out extensive healing and regeneration. Individuals with fibromyalgia spend less time in delta sleep and more time in the lighter phase of sleep, characterized by dreams – often unpleasant.[2,3]

### Fibromyalgia Begets More Fibromyalgia

As with other forms of chronic pain, fibromyalgia is tricky to treat because the condition tends to be self-perpetuating. A healthy body responds to pain and inflammation by initiating regulatory responses to restore equilibrium, thus eliminating the pain and inflammation. However, when pain and stress levels are high enough, they overwhelm the body's ability to regulate itself. A vicious cycle ensues wherein the condition increases in severity like a snowball rolling down a hill. For example:

- The presence of pain interferes with the body's ability to get adequate delta sleep. Therefore, tissue regeneration is compromised, thus worsening the condition.

- Since individuals with fibromyalgia tend to have low energy during the day (from lack of proper sleep at night, perhaps), they often use caffeine and other stimulants to be able to function; this tends to further raise levels of stress hormones, worsening the condition.

- Antidepressants, commonly given for fibromyalgia, disrupt delta sleep.

- As with other chronically painful conditions, individuals with fibromyalgia are less likely to exercise. Exercise increases nitric oxide levels, thus improving oxygenation and overall nutrition of tissues. This in turn, tends to reduce the likelihood of pain and inflammation. Likewise, lack of exercise tends to exacerbate chronic pain.

# Dietary Stressors and Pain

All painful conditions described in this chapter improve when more oxygen is able to reach the tissues. For example, one of the ways in which aspirin reduces pain is by stimulating release of nitric oxide, which dilates local blood vessels. Unfortunately, aspirin, like other pain medications, tends to have harmful side effects. It interferes with the body's ability to repair and regenerate tissues. This is why it causes bleeding or bruising when used regularly.

The good news is that we have other ways to promote nitric oxide production, good circulation, and oxygen utilization by tissues. All the painful conditions described above can improve, sometimes dramatically, with good nutrition. We need only reduce the consumption of stressors that promote pain, while availing ourselves of foods and other nutritional products that help the body to naturally reduce or eliminate pain.

In other words, for many individuals, pain relief might be as simple as making adjustments to their eating habits. In fact, even in cases where food is not the primary cause of pain, dietary adjustments can greatly assist in the elimination or reduction of pain.

## Dietary Stressors that Contribute to Chronic Pain

- **Coffee** contains caffeine, which stimulates the adrenal glands to release stress hormones, contributing to tight muscles.
- **Colas** contain caffeine and other potential stressors, including lots of refined sugar.
- **Alcohol** depletes the body of vitamins, minerals, and other resources, making the individual more susceptible to pain and inflammation.
- **Excess sodium** contributes to tight muscles, irritability, insomnia, swelling, inflammation, joint deposits, and excessive stimulation of the heart.
- **Grains** in excessive amounts can contribute to muscle and joint pain. One of the issues with grains is the presence of gluten, a protein which often triggers allergic reactions. Symptoms of gluten sensitivity include fatigue, abdominal pain, depression, and compromised immune function.  When severe enough, gluten sensitivity can show up on a blood test and is given the medical diagnosis of celiac disease. However, mild (subclinical) intolerance of grains can still contribute to pain and other health issues.
- **Excess protein**, especially of animal origin, can contribute to inflammatory conditions, such as arthritis.[4]
- **MSG** (monosodium glutamate) excites the nervous system, thus contributing to chronically sore muscles. As mentioned in the previous chapter, Dr. Russell Blaylock, a neurosurgeon and author, states that removal of MSG from the diet can eliminate or greatly reduce pain from fibromyalgia. He also suggests that elimination of MSG might be of benefit for individuals with other forms of chronic pain.[5]

**The Issue is Excess**

In the above list of potential stressors, quantity is important, as is quality. Sodium and protein are essential nutrients which are problematical only when overconsumed. Regarding grains, some individuals thrive on properly prepared whole grains as part of a balanced diet. Regarding coffee, a case can be made for its potential benefits, at least for some individuals, as described in Appendix G.

What about alcoholic beverages? Are they okay in small amounts? Perhaps. For some individuals, the presence of other nutrients, such as resveratrol in red wine, could possibly outweigh the negative effects.

MSG is the only item in the above list which most nutritional authorities would agree should be categorically avoided. As described earlier, the concept of a "safe" level of MSG is meaningless because if it is consumed in large enough quantities to change the flavor of food and stimulate the appetite (which is its intended purpose), it will stress the body and potentially kill brain cells. Likewise, colas have no redeeming nutritional qualities, but their toxicity may be said to be less than that of MSG — which isn't saying much.

# Food for Pain Relief

- Many painful conditions can improve when we favor foods that are anti-inflammatory, rich in antioxidants, and rich in nutrients that promote proper oxygenation of tissues. Such foods are listed in chapter 3.

- Stress from any source creates an increased need for omega-3 oils, B vitamins, and especially vitamin C. Ideally, these nutrients should be obtained from whole food sources.

- Malic acid and magnesium, taken together in supplement form, can help reduce the pain and fatigue associated with fibromyalgia.[6]

- Fruits and vegetables can be most helpful in a number of ways. For example, many fruits are rich in malic acid and magnesium. Fruits and vegetables are also the richest source of most vitamins, minerals, and phytonutrients, many of which play a role in reducing inflammation and promoting higher levels of nitric oxide. Furthermore, of all the food groups, fruit provides nourishment in a way that requires the least amount of digestion and cleanup, thus allowing the body to conserve energy which is then available to promote deeper cleansing and healing. The latter point deserves special emphasis because the digestion, clean-up, and repair associated with everyday eating requires a substantial amount of energy and nutrients.

• Freshly made vegetable juice blesses the body in ways similar to fresh fruit. In other words, it is an excellent source of nutrients, in a form that requires little digestion, cleanup and repair. A juice made with kale, apple, fresh ginger, and fresh turmeric can be very helpful in reducing pain and inflammation.

> Many painful conditions can improve when we give the body the nutrition it needs to keep inflammation in check, while optimizing circulation and oxygen utilization.

# Chapter 11
# Strong Bones & Limber Joints

The Key to Skeletal Health
Strong Bones
Limber Joints


Problems with bones and joints are a major reason many individuals limit their physical activity – which then results in further degeneration of the skeleton, as well as the rest of the body. This is how years of eating a less-than-optimal diet, combined with lack of exercise, often create a vicious cycle of physical decline, much of which we assume to be beyond our control, because we perceive it as being part of normal aging. It isn't!

When we awaken to the realization that bones and joints respond beautifully to proper nutrition and exercise, we can then take the appropriate actions. We can literally slow down the aging process, as well as reverse some of the degenerative conditions — including osteoporosis and arthritis.

## The Key to Skeletal Health

The foundation for healthy bones and joints, according to most health authorities, is regular weight-bearing exercise combined with generous helpings of fruits and vegetables, especially leafy greens. Naturally, we also need adequate levels of protein, essential fats, vitamin D, vitamin K and calcium. These too will be addressed in this chapter.

What about skeletal problems due to genetic factors, birth defects, hormonal imbalances, trauma, misaligned bones, or just excessive wear and tear? These other stressors can certainly initiate problems, however, they do not diminish the importance of proper nutrition and exercise. On the contrary, to the extent that skeletal health has been compromised — for whatever reason — good nutrition and proper exercise become that much more important.

# Strong Bones

Osteoporosis (literally, "porous bones"), refers to a loss of bone density, causing bones to become so brittle they can easily break. For example, hip fractures usually occur in older individuals, after years of progressive bone loss.

To prevent or reverse this condition, we must first understand how bones are constructed. Calcium is the most obvious component of bone. Calcium and other minerals make up about 50% of the material making up bone tissue.

Unfortunately, calcium often gets 100% of the attention when a person wants to prevent or reverse osteoporosis. This is a major reason that osteoporosis persists or gets worse even through the person takes a calcium supplement.

To keep bones strong, we must also consider the other 50% bone, which consists mostly of a tough protein called collagen. This is the same collagen that makes up skin, tendons, and ligaments.

Together, collagen and calcium are like the steel and concrete making up a high-rise building. Calcium is the concrete that makes bone rigid. Collagen fibers are like the steel girders in a building; they give bone tensile strength, so it does not crumble when subjected to external forces.

Without collagen, bone tissue would be brittle, like chalk. This is precisely what we see in advanced osteoporosis. More specifically, when an individual gets osteoporosis, both the collagen and calcium content are diminished. If low calcium was the only missing element, the bone would not crumble, it would bend!

The point here is that taking calcium and doing nothing will not correct prevent or reverse osteoporosis. We must address both the collagen and calcium content in order to keep bones strong in younger individuals and reverse osteoporosis in older individuals.

## Common Causes of Osteoporosis

- **Lack of exercise**. Bones are alive. Like muscles, bones respond to exercise by becoming stronger. Exercise promotes both elements of strong bones -- the production of collagen fibers and the deposition of calcium. Likewise, sedentary lifestyle inhibits both processes.
- **Vitamin C deficiency** inhibits collagen production, resulting in loss of tensile strength (brittleness) of bones.
- **Malabsorption of calcium**, often due to lack of vitamin D.

- **Caffeine** contributes to calcium loss. High caffeine intake is associated with increased bone loss and osteoporotic fractures.
- **Soft drinks**, including diet and decaffeinated sodas, are associated with bone loss.
- **Decrease in estrogen**, especially in post-menopausal women, can contribute to bone loss.
- **Anti-inflammatory drugs**, especially cortisone, can accelerate osteoporosis.[1]
- **Oxidative Stress.** Living bone is continuously being built up and torn down. The process of breaking down bone involves free radicals. This might explain why increased oxidative stress is associated with increased bone loss.[2]
- **Milk.** According to worldwide studies, populations with higher dairy consumption is associated with higher rates of bone loss and hip fractures.[3] This puzzling phenomenon was once believed to be due to the strong acidifying influence of the animal protein in milk, leading to removal of calcium from the bones. However, subsequent studies showed that the situation was not that simple. More recent studies suggest that the negative impact of milk on bones mass is probably due to oxidative stress from the galactose (a sugar) in milk.[4]

**The Cure**

Since osteoporosis involves a loss of collagen and calcium, the key to preventing and reversing this condition is to support the body in restoring both.

- **Weight bearing exercises** such as running and resistance training are especially beneficial for promoting strong bones. Exercise stimulates bone cells to make more collagen, while also encouraging the same cells to secret the calcium salts which crystalize around the collagen fibers. With regular exercise, osteoporosis can be reversed, even in elderly individuals. The results are even better when the exercise is combined with proper nutrition.
- **Fruits and vegetables** have been found to promote bone health in both young and old.[5] This is believed to be at least partially due to the high antioxidant content and other factors which downregulates bone breakdown and upregulates bone building.[6]
- **Vitamins D, K** and **C** are important for bone health. Vitamin C is necessary for collagen production. Vitamin D is necessary

for proper absorption of calcium from food. Vitamin K helps keep calcium on the bones.

Vitamin C and vitamin K, are found in fruits and vegetables. In addition, another form of vitamin K (vitamin $K_2$) is produced by some intestinal bacteria. Vitamin $K_2$ is believed to be more potent than the plant derived version. It is available in supplement form.

Vitamin D is best obtained from exposure of the skin to sunshine. However, many individuals don't get enough sunlight to make adequate vitamin D and would therefore benefit from supplementation. Vitamin D and $K_2$, combined into a single supplement, are readily available.

- **Adequate calcium** intake is essential. However, the usual cause of osteoporosis is not lack of calcium. This mineral is easily provided by consuming the same fruits and vegetables that provide vitamin C. Dark green leafy vegetables such as kale and broccoli are excellent sources of calcium.

## Limber joints

A joint is the junction where two or more bones come together. Many painful conditions have to do with joints. Arthritis refers to any inflammatory or degenerative condition of a movable joint.

To understand arthritis and how it can be prevented and possibly reversed, it is helpful to first consider the basic construction of moveable joints. First, to keep friction in check, our bones have a thin layer of smooth glassy cartilage at the point where they come together to form a movable joint. Friction is further reduced by a thick fluid which fills the space between the bones; it is like motor oil lubricating the moving parts of a car's engine. Once we know the basic construction of joint, we can easily understand the three main types of arthritis. They are called osteoarthritis, rheumatoid arthritis and gout.

- **Osteoarthritis** is often called the wear-and-tear arthritis because it is associated with old age or excessive use of joints. The condition is characterized by a decrease in the amount of lubricating fluid between the bones, as well as a thinning of the cartilage on the surface of the bones. Also, the soft tissue associated with the joint, such as the ligaments, may become less flexible and perhaps infiltrated with calcium.

- **Rheumatoid arthritis**, unlike osteoarthritis, has a substantial amount of inflammation, due to an autoimmune attack on joints. Consequently, the cartilage breaks down and scar tissue may bridge the surfaces of the adjoining bones. The scar tissue may become calcified, which means the joint is effectively fused.
- **Gout** is an inflammatory condition resulting from irritating uric acid crystals that accumulate in the joint. High levels of uric acid in the blood are typically the result of large amounts of animal products, especially red meat, in the diet.

**Preventing and Reversing Arthritis**
- Osteoarthritis has been shown to respond well to supplementation with **glucosamine sulfate** — a naturally occurring substance found in joints. It serves as an important building material for cartilage. More specifically, glucosamine sulfate is the key building block for making **chondroitin sulfate**, the substance that makes cartilage what it is – strong and semirigid. In other words, if we think of chondroitin sulfate as a brick wall, the molecules of glucosamine sulfate are the individual bricks. Supplementation with glucosamine sulfate has been shown to decrease joint pain and stimulate regeneration.[7] Some individuals get even better results when the glucosamine sulfate is combined with chondroitin sulfate. Both are readily available in health food stores.

- Adequate **vitamin C** is important for supporting collagen production. Why collagen? Cartilage is not simply made of chondroitin sulfate. Cartilage, like bone, also contains large amounts of collagen.

- **Omega-3 oils** (especially as fish oil or algae oil) has been shown to be beneficial in bringing relief to chronic joint pain.

- **Anti-inflammatory foods** (fruits and vegetables, especially the latter) can be most helpful for both rheumatoid arthritis and gout. Results are even better if we also limit the pro-inflammatory foods (grains, meat, and dairy).

- **Elimination of shellfish and nightshade vegetables** (potatoes, tomatoes, and peppers) can be very helpful for individuals with gout.

- **Reducing animal products** can be helpful with gout. High levels of animal products, especially red meat, will cause the body to make more uric acid, thus irritating gouty joints.

- **Exercise** can help arthritis simply because it can help the body reverse the imbalances that result in pain and inflammation.

- **Aloe Vera** can be helpful in all three forms of arthritis because it helps reduce inflammation and promotes regeneration. It might be especially helpful in rheumatoid arthritis because aloe can help modulate the immune system and reduce autoimmune reactions.[8]

- **Turmeric and ginger**, consumed as freshly squeezed juice or capsules, can be most helpful in alleviating pain from inflamed joints. 2-3 ounces of the juice, diluted with other fluids, might be effective.

# Chapter 12
# Cardiovascular Health

What is a Heart Attack?
The Food Connection
The Heart Healing Diet
To-do List for Cardiovascular Health

The term "life-blood" is appropriate because blood is the bringer of life-giving oxygen and nutrients to our body cells. The same inner current also carries away waste products from our cells. Without blood, our cells would quickly die from lack of nourishment and build-up of cellular excrement.

Blood is propelled by the pumping action of the heart. From the heart, blood circulates through some 60,000 miles of living pipes – arteries, veins, and capillaries.

Arteries convey blood from the heart to all parts of the body. Veins return blood to the heart. Capillaries are microscopic vessels, forming a vast network that channels blood from the tiniest arteries to the tiniest veins.

Our personal river of life starts flowing about three weeks after conception and continues until our time on Earth comes to an end. Indeed, for modern humans, the event that often marks the end of earthly life is the abrupt stopping of our inner river – an event known as a "heart attack."

## What is a Heart Attack?

Cardiovascular disease is still the primary cause of death in industrialized societies. Part of the problem is that cardiovascular problems may develop silently over many years and go completely unnoticed, until the condition is advanced and critical. The first actual sign of such problems is sometimes a fatal heart attack, also known as acute coronary insufficiency, or cardiac arrest. The individual dies because the heart simply cannot pump blood fast enough to keep the person alive.

In other words, when someone dies from cardiac arrest, the problem usually isn't the heart muscle itself, but rather the small coronary arteries that supply the heart. Atherosclerosis is the build-up of fats and fibrous material on the walls of arteries. Such obstructions in the coronary arteries restricts of blood flow, resulting is pain in the chest and left arm.

Prior to the onset of serious symptoms, the individual might get a clue in the form of fatigue after mild exercise, or mild chest and left arm pain after drinking coffee or eating heavily. In males, erectile dysfunction can be an early warning sign for cardiovascular problems. This is due to the fact that erectile issues may result from arterial blockages in the local tissues, which in turn suggests that similar blockages might be present elsewhere — such as the heart.

> Erectile dysfunction can be an early-warning sign for cardiovascular problems.

## What Causes Heart Attacks?

The cause of cardiac arrest is more complicated than once thought. Specifically, it may not be as simple as cholesterol and other materials accumulating in the inner lining of arteries but may have more to do with the rupturing of an arterial plaque, sort of like a pimple spontaneously popping. This, in turn, initiates catastrophic blood clotting reaction that clogs the artery and deprives the heart muscle of blood.[1]

The above finding is important because it suggests that lowering cholesterol (and doing nothing else) will not prevent a heart attack. Indeed, this is precisely what studies have shown: the practice of lowering cholesterol with drugs, while doing nothing else, has not significantly lowered the death rate from cardiovascular disease.[2] Furthermore, cholesterol-lowering drugs have been associated with a number of harmful side-effects[3], such as:

- Memory loss
- Sore muscles, fatigue, and lack of endurance.
- Exercising while on statins is more difficult and post-workout muscle recovery takes longer. This is significant when we consider that exercise can be very effective for reducing cholesterol levels.

A more rational approach is to take steps to prevent or reverse arterial plaquing. We can do this by first understanding how arterial plaque initially forms. Plaquing starts with irritation of the delicate inner lining (endothelium) of the artery. If such irritation exceeds the body's ability to prevent or heal it, chronic low-grade inflammation sets in.

Once inflammation is established, it tends to perpetuate itself, leading to further degenerative changes that include the growth of arterial plaques.[4] As the plaque grows, it progressively diminishes flow of blood in the region, as well as setting the stage for the rupturing of the plaque and catastrophic clotting reaction that blocks the artery.

## The Food Connection

As recently as the 1970s, mainstream medicine did not recognize the connection between diet and cardiovascular health. Prior to that, the idea that cardiovascular problems can be treated with proper diet was dismissed as quackery. Now, the connection between food and heart-health is widely recognized by the medical community. Studies have repeatedly shown that cardiovascular problems can be prevented and reversed through diet.[5, 6]

As described in Chapter 3, chronic low-grade inflammation has been found to be a common thread that triggers many diseases. Since the inflammatory reaction is influenced by food, virtually all degenerative diseases have a dietary connection to some degree.

Pro-inflammatory foods include all foods containing high levels of omega-6 fats, such as corn oil and soy bean oil. In addition, grain-fed beef, dairy, and most grains are pro-inflammatory. Anti-inflammatory foods include fruits, vegetables, and foods rich in omega-3 oils, such as cold-water fish, sea vegetation, and flax seeds.

The eating habits which have been associated with cardiovascular disease typically include too many calories and not enough vitamins, minerals, phytonutrients, and fiber. In other words, the diet has too many pro-inflammatory foods, and not enough anti-inflammatory foods; too many animal products, grains, extracted oils high in omega-6 (safflower and corn oil) and not enough fruits and vegetables.

Below are specific nutritional factors that contribute to arterial plaquing. Notice that inflammation is the key for most of them.

- **Lack of vitamin C** results in loss of integrity of the inner walls of arteries because it is needed to make collagen, which makes up the wall of arteries.[7] (See Appendix H for more details on vitamin C and cardiovascular health.)
- **Deficiency of omega-3 oils** can compromise arteries because these oils are needed to inhibit inflammation and maintain the smoothness and elasticity of the inner lining of blood vessels.[8]
- **Lack of antioxidants.** Much of the damage that leads to inflammation and plaquing is initially caused or accelerated by free-radical damage.[9]
- **Lack of vitamin B12 and folate** can lead to high levels of homocysteine, which irritates the inner lining of blood vessels.[10]
- **Oxidized (heated) oils and trans-fats** can trigger the formation of arterial plaque.
- Diets high in **saturated fats and cholesterol** have been associated with increased risk of cardiovascular disease.[11] However, this is not the same as saying that high levels of these fats *cause* arterial plaquing, as described below.

## Are Saturated Fat and Cholesterol Okay?

Though we would like to have a simple answer to this question, the role of saturated fats and cholesterol in cardiovascular disease is more complex than we used to think. The good news is that we do not need to have all the answers on these fats in order to design a heart healthy diet. One study summarized it as follows:

The role of blood cholesterol levels in coronary heart disease (CHD) and the true effect of cholesterol-lowering statin drugs are debatable. In particular, whether statins actually decrease cardiac mortality and increase life expectancy is controversial. Concurrently, the Mediterranean diet model has been shown to prolong life and reduce the risk of diabetes, cancer, and CHD... We conclude that the expectation that CHD could be prevented or eliminated by simply reducing cholesterol appears unfounded. On the contrary, we should acknowledge the inconsistencies of the cholesterol theory and recognize the proven benefits of a healthy lifestyle incorporating a Mediterranean diet to prevent CHD.[12]

Depending on which dietary philosophy you favor, you might be tempted to interpret the above statement to mean that cholesterol is harmless. However, the authors of the above cited study say no such thing. To properly address the question of causality with regard to cholesterol and cardiovascular disease, we have to be willing to consider the possibility that the answer is not a simple yes or no. Also, for those who have looked into this issue deeply enough to have an opinion, it is important that we free ourselves of the notion that we already know all there is to know about this subject.

Opinions vary as to what constitutes a "healthy level" of saturated fats and cholesterol in food and in the blood. To further complicate matters, the question of individual differences is typically ignored. However, the available data does suggest that we should still go easy on the ingestion of these fats.

## Moderation Still Advisable

Though high levels of saturated fats and cholesterol may not be the primary cause of arterial plaquing, a diet that is high in these fats still contribute to cardiovascular disease in a number of ways. Firstly, high levels of saturated fat in the diet can raise blood cholesterol (specifically LDL cholesterol), which can *speed up* the process of plaque formation, even if it does not actually trigger it. Furthermore, even if we assume that dietary saturated fats and cholesterol do not directly contribute to arterial plaquing, the same diet that is loaded with these fats is likely to have other features that can contribute to cardiovascular disease. For example:

- **Sodium.** The typical diet high in saturated fat and cholesterol also tends to be high in sodium, which tends to stiffen arteries and contributes to high blood pressure, both of which can injure the inner lining of arteries.[13]
- **Oxidized Cholesterol.** Ingesting more cholesterol or having high levels of cholesterol in the blood means that the body will be exposed to more oxidized cholesterol — which has been shown to trigger arterial plaquing. Studies suggest that a relatively small amount of oxidized cholesterol (0.3% of ingested cholesterol) can cause damage to the walls of arteries.[14] A certain amount of oxidized cholesterol is expected in all cholesterol-containing products. More oxidation occurs with cooking, especially at high temperatures, as in broiling, deep-frying, and industrial canning.
- **Heme Iron.** High levels of heme iron can trigger oxidation of cholesterol.[15] Heme iron is found abundantly in red meat.
- Some studies suggest that high blood levels of saturated fats impede dilation of arteries.[16]

- High levels of saturated fats and cholesterol tend to thicken the blood, which tends to increase blood pressure, raise the risk of clot formation, and stresses the delicate inner lining of the blood vessels.
- High levels of dietary saturated fats and cholesterol are associated with insulin resistance. This raises insulin levels which can compromise the integrity of the inner lining of blood vessels. Some studies suggest that a meal high in animal products can raise insulin even more than a plate of pasta.[17]

Bottom line: the available science suggests that dietary saturated fats and cholesterol can be problematic at higher levels. However, a heart-healthy diet must have other features besides appropriate levels of these fats.

## The Heart Healing Diet

Though cardiovascular disease is more complex than once believed, the solution is still rather simple: proper food, proper exercise, and the cultivation of inner peace.

Dietary adjustments have been shown to be effective in preventing and reversing cardiovascular disease. Dietary changes become even more effective when supported by exercise and stress reduction techniques, such as meditation and yoga.[18]

Overall, the carb-based (low-fat) diets have yielded the most consistent results in reversing cardiovascular disease. However, fat-based diets that feature generous portions of fresh produce and plant derived fats such as nuts and seeds have also been used successfully to treat cardiovascular disease.[19, 20] Either way, the key is to make sure the carbs and fats are of the healthy, whole-food variety; with moderate amounts animal products, and ample amounts of fruits and vegetables, especially the latter. A few choice herbs and other nutritional supplements can also be helpful, as described on the next page.

# To-do List for Cardiovascular Health

- Favor foods which are **anti-inflammatory**, rich in **antioxidants,** and rich in nutrients that promote production of **nitric oxide**. These foods are listed on pages 34 and 35.

- Favor a diet that is **moderate in sodium** and **rich in magnesium, potassium,** and **calcium.** This is easily provided by including an abundance of fruits and vegetables.

- Include raw **nuts and seeds,** 1-3 ounces per day, 2-5 times per week. These foods have been associated with lower risk of cardiovascular disease.[21] The protective elements are believed to be polyunsaturated and monounsaturated oils.[22].

- Drink **pomegranate juice.** It contains potent antioxidants that promote vascular health. It also helps to thin blood and reduce blood pressure. Human and animal studies suggest that pomegranate juice can help to reverse atherosclerosis.[23]

- Take **hawthorn berries** in supplement form, or as a tea. Hawthorn berries have been used to treat angina, arrhythmia, high blood pressure and high cholesterol.[24]

- Take **Ginkgo biloba** in supplement form, or as a tea. Ginkgo promotes circulation, as well as thinning the blood.[25] Ginkgo also helps reduce arrhythmias and contains powerful antioxidants that prevent oxidation of LDL cholesterol.

- Drink **hibiscus** tea. Studies suggest that drinking hibiscus can lower blood pressure and cholesterol levels.[26]

- Consider eating **natto,** a form of fermented soy containing nattokinase, which has been shown to thin blood, dissolve clots, and reduce blood pressure.[27]

- Get adequate **omega-3 oils.** These oils reduce inflammation and help maintain the inner lining of blood vessels.

- Get enough **vitamin B$_{12}$** and **folate**. B$_{12}$ is found abundantly in animal products. Folate is found abundantly in leafy vegetables. B$_{12}$ deficiencies are common in the general population, but likely in vegetarians and vegans.

- Take **vitamin E** and **coenzyme Q$_{10}$**. Both are powerful antioxidants as well as supporting the utilization of oxygen by heart cells. Since both are fat soluble, they also act as antioxidants that help prevent oxidation of LDL cholesterol.

- Get enough **vitamin C** and **flavonoids.** In addition to being important to the production of collagen which forms the walls of blood vessels, these nutrients have strong antioxidant activity. As an antioxidant, vitamin C indirectly helps prevent oxidation of LDL cholesterol by restoring the antioxidant power of vitamin E.

  Though the right kind of vitamin C supplement can be of benefit, studies suggest that vitamin C is more effective when obtained from whole foods.[28] For optimum health, around **1000 mg of vitamin C per day** has been suggested. (See Appendix H for a list of foods that are high in vitamin C.)

- **Exercise** promotes cardiovascular health in multiple ways, such as stimulating the release of nitric oxide, which dilates blood vessels.

- Cultivate **emotional poise.** Emotional stress can contribute to the progression of cardiovascular disease in a number of ways. For example, chronic stress tends to thicken the blood and elevate blood pressure, both of which can compromise the health of the heart and arteries. On the neurological level, stress involves sympathetic dominance, which results in depletion of resources and buildup of toxicity – not good for cardiovascular health, as studies have shown.[29]

  In other words, peace and happiness might be as important to cardiovascular health as proper nutrition and exercise. Some would argue that the emotional factors are actually more important than the physical ones. However, I suspect that the heart doesn't argue about such things.

# Chapter 13
# Strong Immune System

The connection between digestion and defense runs deep. For example, one important way that our immune system protects the body from pathogens is through the action of digestive enzymes – the same sort of enzymes used by the digestive system. In other words, enzymes that digest food can also digest diseases.

Beyond the digestive enzyme connection, the digestive system and immune system are deeply connected. Much of what we call immunity is integrated into the workings of the digestive system, with a significant contribution coming from beneficial bacteria in the small and large intestines.

Food is the primary factor determining the quality and quantity of intestinal microbes. Some foods will encourage the growth of beneficial bacteria. Other foods will encourage the growth of the harmful bacteria. Furthermore, foods can influence the immune system in other ways, besides feeding intestinal microbes.

## Digestion and Defense

To better understand the connection between food and the body's defenses, let us first take a closer look at the latter. The body protects itself by two methods: the innate defense and adaptive defense.

**Innate defense**, as the name suggests, is our inborn defense. It responds to all pathogens in pretty much the same way. Our innate defense includes the following:

- *Physical barriers* consist of the skin and mucous membranes. The latter form the inner lining of our air passages and digestive tract.

- *Phagocytosis* is the process by which defensive cells engulf pathogens and dissolve them with digestive enzymes. These cells are found abundantly in and around the digestive tract.
- *Natural killer cells* destroy cancer cells and virus-infected cells. These cells are found abundantly in and around the digestive tract.
- *Beneficial bacteria* in the small and large intestines produce substances that reduce inflammation and support our overall immune response.

**Adaptive defense** is the body's capacity to target specific pathogens. This is done with T and B lymphocytes.
- *T lymphocytes*, also called "T cells," directly attack and destroy specific pathogens.
- *B lymphocytes* produce protein molecules called antibodies in response to specific pathogens. Antibodies protect the body in a number of ways.

After the pathogens have been eliminated, the T and B lymphocytes remain. Therefore, if the same pathogen returns, it is quickly eliminated with little or no discomfort. In this manner, the adaptive defense gives us *immunity* against pathogens encountered in the past. The downside of our adaptive defense is that it can become *mal*adapted.

**Immunity Gone Bad**

In an autoimmune reaction, the body's defenses attack the body's own tissues. Autoimmune diseases include lupus erythematosus, multiple sclerosis, and rheumatoid arthritis.

Many autoimmune diseases are triggered by improperly digested protein which result from eating more protein than the body can comfortably digest. In addition, some types of protein, such as the protein found in dairy, soy, and glutenous grains (wheat, barley, and rye) can be problematic even in moderate amounts.

Apparently Type I Diabetes Meletus can be triggered by an autoimmune reaction. When improperly digested milk protein gets into the blood, the immune system recognizes it as a foreign invader and therefore makes antibodies against it. However, the immune system may not be able to distinguish these foreign proteins from the body's own proteins because the foreign proteins resemble our own. For example, the antibodies may not be able to distinguish dairy protein from the proteins making up the cells in the pancreas which manufacture insulin. As a result, the immune system destroys the insulin-producing cells. This is one of the causes of type I diabetes in young children, as described in Chapter 15.

In addition to the serious autoimmune conditions mentioned above, common allergies may also arise from a poorly functioning immune system. The typical symptoms associated with allergies may include fatigue, headaches, nasal congestion, dark patches under the eyes, asthma, abdominal pain, muscle and joint pain, bladder issues, nervousness, irritability, or feeling "spaced out."

Allergens that cause gastro-intestinal irritation can prevent proper digestion and absorption of nutrients. The subsequent undigested food molecules can then produce more allergic reactions. In other words, immune problems and digestive problems can get locked in a vicious cycle of mutual provocation, causing both to get progressively worse. In addition, all this irritation can ring the adrenal alarm – which brings us back to General Adaptation Syndrome (GAS).

## GAS Revisited

As described in Chapter 9, the body responds to chronic stress from all sources by going into a state called general adaptation syndrome (GAS) wherein the body becomes progressively more depleted and unbalanced. However, the person can have this condition for years without knowing that anything is wrong. In fact, he or she may actually feel better after eating allergens because of the adrenalin rush that follows ingestion of the allergens. Therefore, the body continues to become progressively more unbalanced, until an actual illness occurs, such as fibromyalgia.

A food-craving may signal the presence of allergens. For example, alcoholism typically involves addiction to food derivatives in the beverage – such as wheat, rye, grapes, yeast, or hops. In most cases, it takes about five days to eliminate the effects of an allergen from the body. The individual may initially experience withdrawal symptoms but will eventually feel better.

# Immune System Stressors

- **Foods that stress the immune system** include wheat, corn, soy, coffee, milk, peanuts, chocolate, eggs, tobacco, and beef.
- **Saturated fats and partially hydrogenated vegetable oils.**[1,2] The integrity of cell membranes are influenced by fats making the membranes. When the right kinds of fats are not provided through the foods we eat, the body uses whatever is available.

  Since saturated fats and partially hydrogenated oils are stiffer compared to the omega-3 oils, the result is a reduction in the cell's ability to sense what is happening in its external environment. This can have devastating effects, such as the inability to cope with a virus or other pathogens.
- **Environmental poisons** such as mercury, fluoride, and pesticides tend to inhibit the immune system.[3,4,5]
- **Antibiotics** (see below).

## Antibiotics

Antibiotics are chemicals that disrupt the metabolism of bacteria. Used judiciously, they are a great blessing because they can save a person's life. However, repeated use of antibiotics can produce long-term problems:

- A given antibiotic tends to breed bacterial strains that are resistant to that antibiotic.
- Frequent use of antibiotics tends to weaken the body's defenses. Antibiotics destroy beneficial bacteria which are an important part of our immune system. The body is weakened, thus paving the way for another infection and another round of antibiotics. In other words, the use of antibiotics is, by its very nature, self-perpetuating; repeated use leads to the need for more antibiotics. Furthermore, weening a person off antibiotics may be tricky because the immune system might be compromised to the point of being unable to eliminate infections without strong antibiotics.
- To make matters worse, repeated use of antibiotics can make the body more vulnerable to other conditions besides infections. For example, studies show that individuals with a history of antibiotic-use are more likely to develop colitis and multiple sclerosis.[6,7]

# How to Tune Up the Immune System

Tuning up the immune system means we support it in optimizing its capacity to get rid of pathogens and to do so without harming healthy body tissues. It means we give the body a better chance of getting rid of infections and cancer, as well as reducing the severity of allergic reactions and other autoimmune conditions. Below are some strategies for tuning up the immune system.

- **Keep the Gut Clean and healthy.** A big chunk of our immunity is rooted in the gastrointestinal tract. Therefore, keeping the gut clean and healthy might be the single most powerful way of optimizing the immune system. The other tips given below are effective only to the extent that the gastrointestinal tract is kept clean and healthy.

- Favor foods that are **anti-inflammatory**, rich in **antioxidants** and rich in nutrients that promote the production of **nitric oxide**. These foods are listed on pages 33- 35.

- **Favor colorful fruits and vegetables.** These foods reduce inflammation and free radical damage and support the immune system. For example, blueberries increase the count of natural killer cells, reduce oxidative stress, and increase the production of anti-inflammatory substances in the cells.[8]

- **Take Probiotics**. Since a big chunk of our immunity is rooted in the gastrointestinal tract, with beneficial microbes playing a major role, a probiotic supplement can be helpful, especially after taking antibiotics.

- **Eat Healthy fats.** Favor good sources of omega 3 oil, such as flax, chia seeds, hemp seeds and clean, cold-water fish. Avoid partially hydrogenated vegetable oils.

- **Avoid refined carbohydrates.** These include products made with refined sugar and flour – white bread, cookies, and cakes.

- **Vitamin C** is vital for the immune system. It is best obtained from fresh and raw fruits and vegetables because cooking destroys vitamin C.

- **Elderberry extract** potentizes the immune system against viral infections, especially influenza.[9]

- **Vitamin D** is vital for the immune system. It is best obtained from sunlight which stimulates the skin cells to make vitamin D. Supplementation can be helpful during stressful times or when access to sunlight is limited.

- **Aloe vera** boosts the immune system, reduces inflammation, and has antimicrobial and anti-cancer properties.[10]

- **Olive Leaf Extract** is anticancer, antifungal, antibacterial, and antiviral.[11, 12]

- **Oregano oil** is antiviral antibacterial and antifungal.[13]

- **Rest and Exercise.** The right balance of rest and exercise can go a long way in optimizing the immune system. Exercise is important because the body is simply not designed to be sedentary. Rest is important because it tones down the sympathetic system and activates the parasympathetic system, thus allowing the body to recharge and regenerate.

- **Exercise the Immune System!** As with muscles, the immune system is governed by the principle of "use it or lose it." It becomes strong against pathogens through regular exposure. Granted, hygienic practices have their rightful place. Likewise, social isolation might be appropriate as a temporary measure during times of increased vulnerability. However, overuse of these external measures can weaken the immune system.[14]

- **Cultivate inner peace.** Stress of any kind, especially in the form of depression and fear, can insidiously decimate the immune system over time. Both are very common! An antidote to depression is physical exercise in the great outdoors and loving communion with friends. The antidote to fear is to breathe deeply, go within, and remember the big picture.

### If You Get Sick, Give Thanks!
- Use the illness as an opportunity to correct the internal issues that made you vulnerable to it in the first place.
- In other words, do not just settle for eliminating symptoms and recovering from illness. Go the extra mile!
- Be diligent and follow through with the application of the over strategies, so that you are healthier in body and mind than you were prior to the health challenge.

# Chapter 14
# Cancer Prevention & Treatment

A Man-made Disease
Prevention
Treatment
Diet Options

One of my patients, an older gentleman whom I will call "George," had cancer. He shared with me that he was a farmer in his younger days. Since he was part Native American, he had used traditional farming methods that came down to him from his ancestors. Naturally, they used no pesticides, herbicides, or chemical fertilizers. In addition, they did things to optimize the fertility of the soil. That was how all his farming relatives grew food prior to the 1950s.

In the 1950s, chemical farming became the norm. That was also the beginning of an ever-increasing cancer rate in George's extended family which included numerous aunts and uncles and about 40 cousins. He also said that the 1950s was when cardiovascular disease and diabetes started to become more noticeable in his family.

His medical doctor blamed genetics for the high incidence of cancer and other degenerative diseases in George's family. However, George felt there was more because his grandparents and other relatives from the early 20th century and 1800s did not show the same tendency. In fact, they generally lived to a ripe old age, including some who lived past 100 years.

Eventually, George began to suspect that environmental factors, especially changes in the food supply, may have played a significant role in the high incidence of cancer and other diseases in his family. And that was why he came to see me for nutritional counselling. The information that I shared with him is essentially the information in this chapter.

# A Manmade Disease

As with other illnesses, cancer can have a genetic component.[1] However, a genetic predisposition is much more likely to manifest when environmental triggers are present. Typically, cancer seems to be the result of multiple insults that are leveled against the body by our technology. It is the result of stressors in the form of carcinogens that we have introduced into food, water, and air.[2,3] To this, we may also add other manmade carcinogens in the form of electromagnetic and nuclear toxicity from electronic and mechanical devices.[4] These stressors have proven to be so significant that many health authorities have actively asserted or quietly conceded that cancer is essentially a manmade disease.[5]

The good news is that we can use our technology to cooperate with Nature, rather than trying to conquer it. Food is one of our most powerful resources for preventing cancer. In addition, when intelligently combined with medical and technical knowledge, food can be used in more targeted ways to help eliminate cancer.

In a nutshell, the American Cancer Society, the World Cancer Research Fund, and the American Institute for Cancer Research recommend a diet low in red and processed meats and high in fresh produce — which is similar to the dietary guidelines to protect against diabetes.[6] This is not merely a happy coincidence; it serves as a reminder of an important principle for healing described in chapter 4: any modality that we use to resolve one health issue should at the very least be harmless and ideally of benefit to the rest of the body.

# Prevention

Prevention may seem like a daunting task when we consider the many carcinogens to which we are exposed. However, we don't have to eliminate all of them, or even most of them. When we intelligently address the stressors that are within our power to control, the body will be better able to neutralize the carcinogens that we cannot avoid. This is an important key for disease prevention in general, but it is especially important for a condition like cancer which has a strong environmental component.

> When we take action on stressors we can control, the body will be better able to neutralize stressors that we cannot avoid.

Cancer prevention is about maintaining an internal environment that can accomplish three things:

- Prevents cancer cells from forming in the first place.
- Quickly destroy cancer cells when they do appear.
- Support cleansing and detox.

All three are greatly supported by fruits and vegetables. Their anti-cancer activities are well established.[7] In fact, the variety of fresh produce that has been shown to have cancer-fighting properties is so large that researchers have felt justified in doing studies to compare and catalogue their cancer fighting activity.[8,9,10.] For example, the table below ranks the anticancer activity of commonly consumed fruits and vegetables. The items are listed in the order of decreasing anticancer activity.

| Fruits | Vegetables |
| --- | --- |
| Cranberries | Garlic |
| Lemons | Leaks |
| Apples | Green Onions |
| Strawberries | Brussels Sprouts |
| Red grapes | Cauliflower |
| Grapefruit | Cabbage |
| Bananas | Broccoli |
| Peaches | Radish |
| Oranges | Kale |
| Pineapple | Beets |

As a point of caution, we should bear in mind that the above list is based on just three studies which focused on the most commonly consumed fruits and vegetables. Other studies have shown significant anticancer activity in other forms of fresh produce, as described in the pages that follow.

In general, fruits and vegetables are more potent as health-promoting agents when used in their raw state, but even lightly steamed or sautéed vegetables have benefits.[11] Here are some of the ways that fresh produce can help prevent cancer:

- The fiber and water in fresh produce assist with cleansing and detox. In this case, they help to flush out carcinogens.
- The vitamins, minerals, and phytonutrients in fresh produce serve to potentize the immune system.
- Some phytonutrients directly kill cancer cells or inhibit tumors.

## Cruciferous Vegetables

Studies suggest that cruciferous vegetables have strong anti-cancer properties.[12] These vegetables include broccoli, cauliflower, boc choy, Brussels sprouts, kale, Swiss chard, and collards. Broccoli is the one that has been studied most closely. Its anti-cancer properties seem largely due to the presence of sulfur-containing phytonutrients called glucosinolates.

When broccoli is chopped, blended, or juiced, it releases an enzyme which converts glucosinolates into isothiocyanates (ITCs) – which are especially potent.[13,14,15,16] The conversion does not occur with cooked broccoli because heating food above physiological temperatures destroys enzymes.

## Berries

Research shows that animals whose diets include blackberries and raspberries had a 60% reduction in tumors of the esophagus and up to an 80% reduction in colon tumors.[17] Freeze-dried raspberry powder seemed to normalize the activity of genes that had been altered by a chemical carcinogen.[18]

Blueberries also show promise. In addition to being antioxidant rich, blueberries contain pterostilbene which may help prevent colon cancer. Researchers went so far as to state that this phytonutrient could be developed into a pill with the potential for fewer side effects than some commercial drugs used to prevent cancer.[19] Other studies have shown that blueberries may inhibit breast tumor growth.[20]

## Apples

Apples are rich in health promoting phytonutrients, including polyphenols, flavonoids, procyanidins and anthocyanins. In addition to helping prevent cardiovascular disease, respiratory issues, and diabetes, apples appear to be beneficial for cancer prevention.

Apples are anti-mutagenic and anti-inflammatory. Apples are high in quercetin, a potent anticancer phytonutrient. They show antioxidant activity and epigenetic activation of the immune system.[21] Animal studies suggest that apples can prevent skin, mammary, and colon cancer. German researchers say that drinking two glasses of unfiltered apple juice a day may help prevent colon cancer. Unfiltered apple juice has been found to be up to four times higher in antioxidants than clear apple juice.[22]

## Pomegranates

The wealth of information on the benefits of pomegranates and pomegranate juice for cardiovascular health tends to overshadow their usefulness as anti-cancer agents. The same pomegranate phytonutrients that help to reduce blood pressure and keep the inner lining of arteries flexible and clean, also show promise in fighting cancer. Specifically, the tannins, flavonoids, and polyphenols have been studied for their potential use in cancer prevention and treatment.[23]

## Avocados

Researchers at Ohio University found that avocados stop the uncontrollable growth of pre-cancerous cells that lead to oral cancer. Avocados are also high in lutein and may thus be beneficial in preventing prostate and breast cancer.[24,25] They also have glutathione, an important antioxidant and detoxifier which is believed to be beneficial for preventing cancer.[26]

## Green Tea

Green tea is rich in antioxidants and has been shown to slow down the growth of cancer cells.[27]

## Garlic

According to one meta-analysis (analysis of a number of separate studies), people who consume garlic regularly have about half the risk of stomach cancer and two-thirds the risk of colorectal cancer as those who eat little or none.[28]

## Turmeric

Turmeric has received much attention in recent years for its multiple health benefits, largely due to its powerful antioxidant and anti-inflammatory activities, both of which are important in cancer prevention and treatment.[29]

# Treatment

As with prevention, a rational strategy for treating cancer should include methods that support the body in three ways:

• Directly kill cancer cells and inhibit tumor growth.
• Indirectly kill cancer cells by potentizing the immune system.
• Support cleansing and detox.

The last bullet point is easy to overlook when the individual has a rapidly growing tumor that must be eliminated as quickly as possible. Under such circumstances, the main focus is on surgery, powerful drugs and/or radiation to directly kill cancer cells. However, studies suggest that such methods of direct frontal attack are more likely to produce good long-term results if the body is supported with foods and nutritional products that facilitate general cleaning and detoxification, as well as enhancing the immune system.[30]

In addition to being exposed to specific carcinogens, cancer patients are often in a general state of toxicity, as well as having a number of deficiencies. Strong chemotherapy drugs and radiation only add to the toxic burden. Therefore, common sense tells us that the same foods associated with cancer prevention should also have a place in cancer treatment.

## Correcting Toxicity and Deficiencies

Cancer patients are typically deficient in vitamins, minerals, and phytonutrients. Among their many roles, these nutrients often serve as antioxidants, which are important for preventing cancer. Therefore, common sense suggests that such nutrients should be included in the cancer patient's nutritional regimen. These nutrients are best obtained from whole foods.

The richest sources of antioxidants are fresh and raw produce. Raw fruits and vegetables are also the most cleansing of foods. Their low toxicity and high levels of water and fiber facilitate removal of waste products and other chemical irritants from the body. More and more health care practitioners are advising cancer patients to favor these foods.

## Vegetables and Their Juices

Vegetables and their juices are used liberally in alternative cancer treatments. The most commonly used vegetables are carrots, beets, cruciferous vegetables, and dark leafy green vegetables.[31] In addition, to being rich in micronutrients, they are also the most alkalizing of foods.[32]

Why should we juice vegetables? Since the body's capacity to digest and absorb nutrients is often compromised in cancer patients, alternative cancer treatments often take special measures to infuse the body with large amounts of needed nutrients without overtaxing the digestive system. In that regard, juicing is ideal because it concentrates micronutrients and makes them available in a form that is easily absorbed. This can be a great blessing for a body that has been depleted by chronic stress or illness.

For cancer patients, juicing is especially beneficial when raw cruciferous vegetables are included. The previously described ITCs in cruciferous vegetables have been shown to actually kill cancer cells, as well as remove carcinogens and detoxify the body. However, in order to convert glucosinolates into ITCs, the cell walls of the vegetables must be broken down. A powerful juicer can do this more effectively than chewing. Juicing also concentrates ITCs to potentially therapeutic levels.

## Microgreens and Their Juices

Microgreens are the seedlings of common plants, such as wheat, barley, cilantro, peas, broccoli, and sunflower. They are grown in soil and usually harvested within two weeks of planting, at which time they might contain up to *40 times* higher levels of key nutrients compared to the mature plant. They are especially rich in nutrients when grown on mineral rich soil, such as mushroom compost or worm castings. For example, the level of ITCs in broccoli sprouts and microgreens is much higher than mature broccoli. Therefore, juiced broccoli sprouts or microgreens can make a potent ITC cocktail, as suggested by some researchers.[33, 34]

## Blended Vegetables

Though juicing is useful for getting concentrated micronutrients into a depleted body, some fiber is still needed. This is where a powerful blender can be used to liberate nutrients in a manner similar to juicing, while still retaining the fiber.

However, we should emphasize that blending does not replace juicing, because it cannot concentrate micronutrients as much as juicing. Blending simply offers a way of bringing the benefits of fiber into the diet in a way that reduces the workload on the digestive system.

## Foods High in Carotenoids

Carotenoids are found in many vegetables and fruits. They are responsible for the bright yellow to orange color of carrots, sweet potatoes, and papaya. Some carotenoids such as beta-carotene are converted into vitamin A. Many have strong antioxidant activity, as well as supporting the immune system. Studies suggest that a diet high in carotenoids would benefit cancer patients.[35]

**Fruit**

Some students of nutrition have assumed that sugar in whole fresh fruit contributes to tumor growth. They therefore conclude that fruit should be restricted for the cancer patient. This idea is based on the observation that sugar does indeed feed cancer cells. However, the assumption about fresh fruit promoting tumor growth ignores the simple fact that blood sugar (glucose) feeds *all* our body cells — as do protein and fat! All three nutrients are essential to maintain health. All three consumed in excess promote tumor growth.

Any confusion regarding sugars, fats, and protein feeding cells quickly clears up when we take a closer look at the word, "feed." How exactly do sugars, fats, and protein feed cancer cells? They do so in the same way that they feed *all* body cells: sugars are used mostly as fuel, which means they are burned for energy. In contrast, protein and fat provide most of the building materials, which means they are assembled into the very fabric making up cells and tissues. The problem with all three nutrients arises through excess! The right amount of sugars, fat, and protein feed healthy body cells. Too much of the same three nutrients feed the tumor, each in their own way.

Furthermore, the assumption that fruit is bad for cancer patients flies in the face of numerous studies which show that fresh fruit contains a wealth of nutrients known to help the body prevent and reverse tumor growth. Apples, blueberries, blackberries, and raspberries are just a few of the fruits that show promise in cancer prevention and treatment. For example, resveratrol, found in red and purple grapes and red wine, has been shown to kill cancer cells.[36] Red grapes are also rich in quercetin, another anticancer phytonutrient. Sweet fruits often produce polyphenols that protect them from fungus and have the added effect of killing cancer cells.[37] However, the use of fungicides seems to suppress the production of these cancer fighting agents. This is yet another reason to favor organic and naturally grown fruits and vegetables.

Even when the importance of phytonutrients in fruit is recognized, some health practitioners assume that such nutrients are best consumed in the form of isolated extracts so as to increase potency and eliminate the supposedly harmful fruit sugars. However, research shows otherwise. For example, some anti-cancer drugs work best when accompanied by glucose. For the same reason, they work better in the presence of insulin because it expedites absorption of glucose by cells. Essentially, when the cancer cells open up to let the glucose in, they also get a mouthful of the anti-cancer substance.[38,39]

Similarly, studies suggest that cancer-fighting nutrients in fruit often require the presence of the fruit sugars to work at an optimum level. For example, the ellagic acid in berries, and resveratrol in red and purple grapes, are absorbed more readily by cancer cells in their whole food form.

Here is a quote from D. Nixon MD, who researched the cancer fighting properties of ellagic acid in raspberries: "What is interesting to note is the superior efficacy of eating red raspberries as opposed to taking the individual phytochemicals in the form of dietary supplements."[40]

## Integrated Cancer Treatment

The nutritional options presented above do not preclude the possibility of using conventional medical treatment. In the past, some oncologists expressed concern that using nutritional support during chemotherapy or radiation might interfere with medical treatment by "protecting" the cancer cells. This seems like a legitimate concern but the reality of it is the opposite. As mentioned earlier, the use of nutritional support during cancer treatment tends to reduce adverse reactions to the medical treatments while improving the overall long-term results. One study showed that resveratrol, among its many benefits, protects normal tissues from the adverse effects of chemotherapy while rendering the cancer cells more vulnerable to the drug.

Another form of integrated cancer treatment that shows promise involves the use of proteolytic enzymes along with chemotherapy drugs. The reason? Tumors generally coat themselves with a protein called fibrin. This is why cancer researchers doing in-vitro investigations of chemotherapy drugs often bathe cancer cells in proteolytic enzymes. The enzymes dissolve the protein coat, thus exposing the cancer cell surface to the drug. This might be one reason that a drug that works well in-vitro might perform poorly in the body.[41] This might also explain why the body's own immune system is often unable to break down a tumor in the first place!

Not surprisingly, some forms of alternative cancer treatment use proteolytic enzymes to dissolve the fibrin coat to expose cancer cells to the immune system. Until recently, this practice was not officially recognized by mainstream medicine. This seems to be changing because studies are emerging which show that the use of such enzymes, along with the usual chemotherapy drugs, demonstrate that enzyme therapy can increase the patient's response rate, duration of remission and survival rate, as well as reducing the side effects from the drugs.[42]

Is there any benefit to eating foods that are naturally high in proteolytic enzymes? As of this writing, we have no hard evidence to support this idea, but it is certainly worth a try — since the person has to eat anyway! Obviously, such high-enzyme foods should be eaten raw because cooking destroys enzymes

Three foods that are especially high in proteolytic enzymes are pineapple, papaya, and kiwi. Even if the therapeutic value from their enzymes turns out to be minimal, these same foods are also very high in vitamin C and various phytonutrients which are of great value to the cancer patient.

Another form of integrated cancer treatment currently being investigated is the use of short-term fasting, along with chemotherapy. In addition to slowing down tumor growth, fasting and caloric restriction seem to cause normal cells to shift into a protective mode wherein they become more resistant to the harmful effects of chemotherapy drugs. In contrast, cancer cells become *more* vulnerable during a fast![43]

# Diet Options

The overall dietary strategy for supporting a cancer patient has two essential features:

- Keep calories on the low side, especially in the form of protein.
- Include foods that provide generous amounts of vitamins, minerals, phytonutrients, and fiber.

The reason to be modest with calories is that cancer, like virtually all degenerative diseases, thrives on surplus calories. In this case, surplus calories translate into extra fuel which cancer cells can burn for energy, as well as providing extra building material to make new cancer cells.

The reason to single out protein for reduction is that it is the main building material for all body cells. Therefore, an abundance of protein is needed by any rapidly growing tissue – such as cancerous tissue.

On the other hand, an abundance of micronutrients and fiber provide the following benefits which greatly support the body in eliminating cancer.
- Strengthen the immune system
- Alkalize the body
- Promote detoxification
- Reduce inflammation
- Allow for proper oxygenation of cells

Beyond the overall strategy given above, the two basic options for an anti-cancer diet are either carb-based or fat-based. The great news is that both dietary options can be easily adjusted so they do not support the spreading of cancer, and possibly play a significant role in eliminating it.

### Fat-Based (low-carb) Diet

The main rationale for using this sort of diet is that carbohydrate intake will be low, thus depriving cancer cells of fuel to burn for energy. Granted, some types of cancer can and do burn fat and even protein for energy, but cancer cells generally burn glucose as their default fuel.

One version of this diet, the **ketogenic diet**, has gotten much attention because it seems to be effective in helping to shrink some tumors. There are three possible reasons for this:

- Since carbs are kept very low, cancer cells are deprived of the fuel they need to generate energy. With insufficient energy, cancer cells have a hard time replicating.
- According to some studies, the ketone bodies which are generated with this diet appear to inhibit tumor growth.[44]
- The same very low carbohydrate levels which deprive cancer cells of energy may also trigger breakdown of the body's own protein – which ordinarily should be avoided, but in this case, can be therapeutic. You see, when the body is forced to burn its own protein for energy, it will tend to cannibalize the *most expendable* protein first – such as the protein that forms tumors and their fibrous covering!

### Carb-Based (low-fat) Diet

The carb-based diet restricts fat and protein. It does not restrict carbohydrates per se' but does avoid their overconsumption as part of the general strategy of being modest with total calories. The reasons why the carb-based approach might be effective are as follows:

- By keeping both protein and fat low, tumors are deprived of the brick and mortar they need to grow. This sort of diet often eliminates all animal protein — which are typically dominated by fat and protein.
- By minimizing animal products, cholesterol is also eliminated. High levels of cholesterol stimulate tumor growth because it is a key building material for rapidly reproducing cancer cells.
- As part of the strategy of avoiding caloric excess, concentrated carbs, as in grains and potatoes, are reduced. They are replaced with fresh fruits and vegetables, which have far fewer calories but more fiber and cancer fighting micronutrients.
- With animal products restricted, methionine and leucine are reduced, thus inhibiting reproduction of cancer cells. Methionine is an amino acid which is needed by all body cells. However, cancer cells are especially sensitive to low levels of this amino acid; they are unable to multiply and become more vulnerable to anti-cancer agents.[45] In that regard, fruit is ideal because it is very low in methionine.

The **NORI Protocol** is one version of the carb-based diet that specifically restricts the amino acid methionine.[46] This plan uses fruits and vegetables liberally, while avoiding foods that offer higher levels of methionine, such as meat, dairy, and grains. In addition, after cancer cells have been weakened by low methionine levels, natural anti-cancer agents are used to destroy them.

Like the ketogenic diet, the Nori Protocol and other such low-fat diets should be done under proper supervision so the individual can be closely monitored. In addition, the developer of the NORI Protocol states that the diet works best when tailored to the individual, rather than using the same exact protocol for very patient.

# Chapter 15
# Stable Blood Sugar

A Baffling Illness
Diabetes Mellitus
How the Body Regulates Blood Sugar
Diets for Diabetes
Tips for Regulating Blood Sugar

"How many of you know someone who has diabetes?" This is a question I have often asked while teaching a Nutrition or Anatomy & Physiology class. Over the years, the number of students who raise their hands has increased significantly. In the U.S., diabetes mellitus is currently the seventh leading cause of death.[1]

Many individuals may have blood sugar problems without realizing it. In addition, those who do know it may not be aware that food can make a huge difference. Moreover, until recently, blood sugar problems were baffling to medical doctors.

## A Baffling Illness

Carbohydrates in food become blood sugar. That part of the blood sugar puzzle is straightforward. Therefore, the solution to blood sugar problems seemed to be to lower dietary carbohydrates. However, this strategy did not produce the expected results in a consistent manner; and for most of the 20th century, no one knew why. Medical doctors simply continued raising the dosage of insulin, as the patient's health continued to deteriorate.

The good news is that we now know enough about blood sugar regulation to address this condition more effectively. As a point of caution, however, we still cannot claim to know all there is to know about this subject. Emerging data suggests that blood sugar regulation is more intricate than we used to think.[2]

To understand why blood sugar problems were so baffling in the past, let us first consider what we do know about blood sugar regulation. In so doing, we will also be setting the stage for understanding how to stabilize blood sugar.

# How the Body Regulates Blood Sugar

Our blood sugar is glucose. It serves as fuel which our cells burn for energy. Since blood glucose is continuously absorbed and burned by our body cells, it must be replenished. The source of new glucose is food. Glucose can come directly from sweet foods, such as fruit, but more typically comes from starchy and semi-starchy foods, such as grains, beans, potatoes, and winter squash.

A starch molecule is simply thousands of glucose molecules linked together like beads on a string. When starch is digested in the gut, it is broken down into many glucose molecules.

Molecule of glucose: 0
Molecule of starch:  0—0—0—0—0—0—0—0—0—etc.

Whether glucose is derived from dietary sugars or starches, it is eventually absorbed by our cells where it is burned for energy or stored for later use.

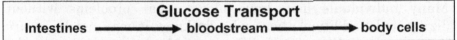

**Glucose Transport**
Intestines ⟶ bloodstream ⟶ body cells

## Blood Sugar and Insulin

The primary hormone for regulating blood-sugar is insulin which is produced by the pancreas. Insulin decreases blood glucose by promoting its absorption by body cells. Not surprisingly, when large amounts of glucose enter the blood from the gut, the pancreas releases extra insulin, causing cells to absorb the extra glucose. The cells burn enough of it to meet their immediate energy needs. Any surplus is handled in one of two ways:

• Glucose is stored as glycogen in the liver and muscles.
• Glucose is transformed into body fat.

## The Overworked Pancreas

The pancreas is overtaxed when the amount of glucose entering the bloodstream exceeds the body's ability to gracefully move it into the cells. This glucose log-jam can occur for one of two reasons:

•Too much glucose enters the blood-stream from the gut.
• Our cells' ability to absorb glucose has been compromised.

**Impaired Glucose Transport**
Gut ⟶ bloodstream ⟶ body cells

Historically, most of the medical attention was focused on limiting the rate at which glucose enters the blood. This was done by restricting carbohydrates in the diet. However, this seemingly logical strategy did not address the cells' impaired ability to absorb glucose from the blood. This is the main reason that the standard dietary guidelines of the past did not produce the expected results.

Looking at the bigger picture, whether ingested glucose is excessive, or the cells' ability to absorb glucose is impaired, the result is the same – either way, blood sugar levels become too high. Consequently, the pancreas has to produce extra insulin.

To complicate matters, if the surge of insulin is great enough, it can pull *too much* glucose into the body cells, resulting in blood glucose levels dropping too low. This is when the individual might feel the urge to eat more sugary foods — which, in turn, triggers another big release of insulin. If this is repeated habitually, the individual develops hypoglycemia, a condition of chronically low blood sugar.

The symptoms of hypoglycemia are fatigue, "brain fog," irritability, depression, moodiness, and craving of sweets. The latter obviously leads to more sugar intake, which in turn worsens the condition. Eventually, hypoglycemia can progress to diabetes mellitus.

## Diabetes Mellitus

Diabetes mellitus is a condition characterized by chronically high levels of glucose in the blood. The diagnosis is based on two blood tests: fasting blood sugar and hemoglobin A1C.[3] Since glucose is essentially stalled in the blood and cells are not properly nourished, widespread health issues may occur, such as blindness, slow wound healing, and ulcers.

In addition, the body responds to the lack of glucose in the cells by putting more fat into the blood, which increases the likelihood of atherosclerosis. Extra glucose in the blood also causes it to pass out through the urine, along with extra water, resulting in increased urine production. Not surprisingly, a person with diabetes produces copious amounts of urine. Therefore, the individual either drinks a lot of water or experiences chronic dehydration.

## Two Types of Diabetes

To effectively treat diabetes mellitus, we must first understand the two major types.[4,5]

- **Type I diabetes** is a condition in which the pancreas does not produce adequate amounts of insulin. This condition was formerly called "juvenile diabetes" because it typically occurred in children. For many years, type 1 diabetes was assumed to be entirely genetic. However, the genetic predisposition seems to require a trigger – food. Apparently, certain foods can induce an autoimmune reaction wherein the insulin-producing cells in the pancreas are destroyed. This can happen in response to the chronic ingestion of allergens, most notably dairy.[6]

- **Type II diabetes** is characterized by *insulin resistance*, wherein the body cells become "numb" to the presence of insulin. Type II used to be called "adult-onset diabetes," because, in the past, a person had to be well into adulthood before the body succumbed to this condition. Not so anymore. Its increased presence in children coincides with a sharp rise in childhood obesity – which comes as no surprise when we consider the increased consumption of fast food and decrease in physical activity. Since type II diabetes accounts for 90% of diabetic individuals, let us take a closer look at insulin resistance.

### Insulin Resistance

When the body cells become numb or resistant to the presence of insulin, the pancreas has to secrete more insulin in order to illicit a response from the cells. Eventually, the pancreas becomes exhausted, insulin levels drop, and blood sugar levels rise rapidly to diabetic levels. This is why years of hypoglycemia often leads to diabetes.

### Side Effects of High Insulin Levels

Besides causing blood sugar issues, insulin resistance has other serious long-term consequences. Since the cells are numb to the presence of insulin, the pancreas is forced to produce higher levels of this hormone, which harms the body in a number of ways:

- High insulin levels inhibit the secretion of growth hormone and thereby   accelerates tissue degeneration.
- High insulin levels stimulate arterial plaquing.
- High insulin levels interfere with the removal of cholesterol from the blood.

- High insulin levels damage kidneys.
- High insulin levels damage the retina of the eyes.

Here are the major dietary and lifestyle factors that tend to reduce our cells' insulin sensitivity.

- **Lack of Exercise**. Physical activity has a profound positive impact on insulin sensitivity. The more we exercise, the greater the insulin sensitivity. Likewise, sedentary lifestyle greatly reduces insulin sensitivity.

- **Dehydration** makes body cells more resistant to insulin, which eventually leads to an increase in blood sugar.[7] When blood glucose is high enough, it escapes through the urine. The presence of glucose in the urine results in greater water loss from the body, thus contributing to more dehydration, which further increases insulin resistance, and so on. In other words, insulin resistance and dehydration can form a vicious cycle, wherein each contributes to the progression of the other.

- **Stimulants.** Blood sugar problems can manifest as fatigue. Individuals who are chronically tired often compensate by taking stimulants which cause the adrenal glands to secrete higher levels of stress hormones, most notably cortisol. Chronically high cortisol levels can increase insulin resistance. This is another vicious cycle that can accelerate the progression of blood sugar issues.

    Caffeine is a common stimulant which can contribute to insulin resistance. MSG is another stimulant that is often consumed without the person knowing it because it is used in processed foods and restaurants – especially fast food.

    In addition to ingested stimulants, any other stressor that over-stimulates the adrenal glands, including emotional stress and lack of sleep, can contribute to insulin resistance and blood sugar issues.

- **Excess carbohydrates** can destabilize blood sugar in two ways: First, they can exhaust the pancreas. Secondly, before the pancreas is exhausted, it produces high levels of insulin, which can lead to insulin resistance. The typical sources of chronic carbohydrate surplus are refined foods, usually white bread, and refined sugar. However, the effect that a given amount of carbohydrates has on blood sugar depends on other factors, such as the amount of protein and fat in the same diet.

- **Excess Protein.** High levels of protein can contribute to insulin resistance because protein triggers insulin release – just like carbohydrates.[8] Higher levels of insulin, by any means, can contribute to the cells becoming less sensitive to it. Studies suggest that protein from animal sources are more problematic than plant protein in this regard.[9] This may be due, at least in part, to the presence of heme iron in animal products, which can adversely affect blood sugar regulation.[10]

  Animal protein has also been shown to raise levels of IGF-1 (insulin-like growth factor-1), which has been linked with type II diabetes — as well as cancer, cardiovascular disease, rapid aging, and reduced lifespan.[11]

- **Excess Fat.** High levels of body fat and dietary fat reduce insulin sensitivity. A number of studies show that high levels of fat in the body cells and blood stream slow down the absorption of glucose by our body cells. [12,13,14,15]

  In one study, subjects were given an abundance of fatty foods. Within two days, their blood sugar elevated to diabetic levels.[16] In another study, a burger's worth of beef or three slices of cheddar cheese boosted insulin levels more than two cups of cooked pasta.[17] In contrast, low-fat (high-carbohydrate) diets, done properly, seem to be effective in managing or reversing diabetes, at least in some individuals.[18,19]

  Saturated fats, omega-6 fats (most vegetable oils), and trans-fats seem to be especially problematic. Studies show that high levels of saturated fats in cell membranes are linked to an increase in insulin resistance.[20] On the other hand, omega-3 fats have been shown to promote insulin sensitivity. Omega 3 fats have been shown to decrease blood sugar levels in diabetics.

To complete the fat picture, as a point of caution, we must also add that the studies linking higher levels of fat with blood sugar problems usually do not account for the protein and carbohydrates in the same diet. This is an important point because the mixing of high-fat, high-carbohydrate, and high-protein foods is very common. This is true for fast foods, as well as meals that might be considered "healthy." Carbohydrates can have a profound effect on how a fat-rich diet effects blood sugar, as described below.

## Double Whammy

Fats and carbs can clash if both are present in large amounts in the same diet, and especially in the same meal. This is not surprising; when we consider that high levels of both carbs and fats do not occur in a given naturally-occurring foods.

Typically, whole foods provide the bulk of calories from carbohydrates, with much lower levels of fats, or vice versa. For example, meat, poultry, and fish provide the bulk of calories from fat, with virtually no carbohydrates. Likewise, nuts and seeds provide the bulk of calories from fat, with much lower levels of carbohydrates. On the other hand, grains, beans, fruits, and vegetables provide the bulk of calories from carbohydrates, with much lower levels of fat.

When our ancestors learned how to store and cook food, they began mixing high-fat with high-carb foods. For example, cookies, cakes, sweet breads, ice-cream, pizza, baked potatoes with sour cream or butter, potato chips, French fries, and turkey sandwiches are typically made by combining concentrated sources of carbohydrates (such as wheat flour and refined sugar), with fats (vegetables oils, shortening or butter). Such combinations can result in digestive disturbance and impaired glucose regulation, even when the ingredients consist of high-quality whole foods. It is a safe bet that the typical individual with type II diabetes got that way by chronically over-consuming foods that have both high levels of carbohydrates and fats. This is why the practice of food combining is often used to correct health problems.

Food combining guides the individual in avoiding the mixing of large amounts of carb-rich foods with large amounts of fatty foods. This is why virtually all diets are either "low-carb" or "low-fat." Both have been used successfully to help stabilize blood sugar.

## Fruit and Blood Sugar

Many dietary authors advise moderation or even total abstinence of fruit for individuals with blood sugar issues. This seems logical, but here again, we must apply this logic within the context of the bigger picture:

- The usual alternatives to fruit as a source of carb-calories, are cooked starchy vegetables and grain products which often have a higher glycemic index than most raw fruits. The glycemic index is a measure of how quickly a food sends glucose into the blood (see Appendix I).

- Most fruits are middle or low glycemic. The only fresh fruits that border on high glycemic are watermelon and grapes.

- Fruits offer benefits that often outweigh the glycemic index. For example, pomegranate has a glycemic index of 67, which is on the high end of medium glycemic, but also contains phytonutrients in the juice and the seeds that help regulate blood glucose. Grapes are another example of a fruit that is high in sugar but also has phytonutrients that lower blood sugar. In the latter case, the active ingredients are found in grape skin and have actually been extracted and marketed for that purpose, as well as providing other benefits.[21]

- Studies done on individuals eating a high-fruit diet have shown no adverse effects on blood sugar, insulin levels, cholesterol, triglycerides, and blood proteins, and in some cases showed beneficial changes in these markers.[22,23]

- Fruits have soluble fiber which helps to stabilize blood sugar, as described below.

## Fiber and Blood Sugar

Plant fiber slows down the passage of sugars into the blood. Soluble fiber is especially helpful with blood sugar regulation. One form of the fiber in fruit is called pectin, a soluble fiber that is soft and absorbent. Soluble fiber is also found in some vegetables, grains, legumes, and seeds.

# Diets for Diabetes

The American Diabetic Association recommends an individualized approach in which the person favors either a carb-based diet, or a fat-based diet rich in monounsaturated fats.[24] In other words, get the bulk of your daily calories from carbs, while keeping fats on the low side, or vice versa.

Carbohydrates, by their very nature, necessitate secretion of insulin. As the level of carbohydrates in the diet increases, the pancreas must secrete more insulin. Meanwhile, fats, in substantial amounts, tend to slow down the absorption of glucose by our cells. Therefore, common sense suggests that the individual with diabetes would do well to avoid having both fats and carbohydrates in substantial amounts.

## Carb-Based Diet

Carb-based diets featuring whole foods with an abundance of fresh produce have been shown to be effective in reversing diabetes.[25] Yes, the carbs are high, but if fats are low and the rest of the diet and lifestyle promote insulin sensitivity, the body is able to manage the carbs very nicely, without overtaxing the pancreas.

In a carb-based diet, the staple foods are typically grains, starchy vegetables, and legumes. Legumes have been associated with reduced risk of diabetes.[26] Modest amounts of nuts and seeds (1-3 ounces, several times per week), can also be beneficial. [27]

## Fat-Based Diet

Some diabetic individuals seem to respond more favorably to a fat-based diet.[28] Yes, fats tend to slow down absorption of glucose by the body cells. However, if total dietary carbohydrates are low and all the other glycemic ducks are in a row, insulin sensitivity can still be maintained at a level that allows for proper regulation of blood sugar, without overtaxing the pancreas.

Diabetics on a fat-based diet are advised to favor plant fats with a good amount of monounsaturated fats, as suggested by the American Diabetes Association. Diabetics are also advised to include foods that provide omega-3 oils, such as flax seeds, hemp seeds, and chia seeds.

At the time of this writing, one researcher was exploring an innovative fat-based diet which uses mostly plant-derived fats and modest amounts of animal products. What makes this plan unique is that it carefully maintains the carbohydrate/protein ratio at 3.65 to 1. The researcher states that this specific ratio appears to help patients with blood sugar issues who are also susceptible to cognitive decline, mood swings, and physical weakness. [29]

Animal foods such as cold-water fish and free-range eggs can still be used. One benefit of including such animal products is long-chain omega-3 fats (EPA and DHA) which promote insulin sensitivity, as well as providing other benefits. However, the use of eggs by diabetics remains controversial. Some studies link eggs to insulin résistance, while others suggest that eggs might *improve* insulin sensitivity for individuals who also limit their carb intake.[30.] Moderation with eggs is still advisable because diabetics seem to be more susceptible to elevated blood cholesterol from ingesting cholesterol.[31] The egg controversy is described in more detail in Appendix A.

# Tips for Regulating Blood Sugar

- Stay **well hydrated.** Hydration promotes insulin sensitivity.

- **Exercise regularly.** Physical activity is as important as proper nutrition for maintaining optimal insulin sensitivity.

- **Favor anti-inflammatory foods** rich in **antioxidants** and rich in nutrients that promote the release of **nitric oxide.** These foods are listed on pages 33 to 35.

- **Emphasize low-starch vegetables,** especially the leafy kind. Veggies provide a wealth of vitamins, minerals, phytonutrients, and fiber, all of which are essential for blood sugar regulation [32]

- **Include whole fruit** in the diet. Like vegetables, fruit provides a wealth of vitamins, minerals, phytonutrients, and fiber that play a role in maintaining proper blood sugar.[33] Fruit has been associated with decreased risk of diabetes.[34]

- **Favor low glycemic fruit**. Though most fruits are middle to low glycemic, common sense suggests that the individual with diabetes should favor lower glycemic fruits, such as berries, kiwi, and cherries. I would also suggest adjusting the amount of fruit in accordance with your needs, rather than arbitrarily relying on a one-size-fits-all formula. For most diabetics, 2-4 servings of fresh fruit per day is safe and beneficial. However, use your common sense and your life experience to up-regulate or down-regulate fruit consumption to fit your personal needs.

- **Avoid trans-fats,** as in margarine and shortening.

- **Avoid refined sugars and white flour.**

- **Be moderate with high-calorie foods**, especially extracted oils and "healthy" cookies, cakes, and pies. Regulate portions so as to leave room for fresh produce.

- **Consume raw nuts and seeds**, especially those with higher levels of omega 3 oils, such as chia, hemp, and flax seeds. Flax seeds are also rich in soluble fiber.

- **Consume animal products in moderation.**[35,36,37] The effect of eggs on insulin sensitivity seems to depend on the individual's overall diet.

| Foods and Supplements for Blood Sugar Regulation | |
| --- | --- |
| Alpha-lipoic Acid | Encourages the absorption of glucose by body cells. |
| N-Acetyl Cysteine | Encourages the absorption of glucose by body cells. |
| Coenzyme $Q_{10}$ | Lowers blood sugar and promotes proper utilization of glucose and oxygen. |
| Omega-3 oils | Promote insulin sensitivity. |
| Chromium | Promotes insulin sensitivity. |
| Zinc | Promotes production of insulin. |
| Cinnamon | Promotes insulin sensitivity and works with insulin to lower blood glucose. |
| Bitter Melon | Reduces insulin resistance. |
| Pomegranates, berries, cucumber, spinach, broccoli, Brussels sprouts, asparagus | Contain soluble fiber, as well as phytonutrients and oils that enhance insulin sensitivity. |

# Chapter 16
# Yeast & Other Fungal Conditions

The Fungus Among Us
Foods that Feed Fungus
Foods to Eliminate Fungus
The Candida Cleanse
How to Make Cultured Vegetables

The health problems associated with fungal infestation can include fatigue, urinary tract infections, vaginitis, gas, bloating, depression, "brain fog," skin rashes, psoriasis, hives, runny nose, headaches, itching and burning in the groin area and feet, rotting toenails, and just feeling bad all over.

## The Fungus Among Us

The specific yeast that can proliferate systemically as well as the gastrointestinal tract and vagina, is called Candida albicans. Other common fungal conditions include ringworm, thrush, jock itch, athlete's foot and toenail fungus. All of them feed on sugars. Therefore, if we properly address one fungal issue – by taking away its food supply – the others, if present, are likely to improve as well.

A certain amount of Candida in the gastrointestinal tract is normal. However, certain stressors create an internal environment that permits yeast to overgrow and eventually colonize other parts of the body such as the brain, kidneys, and heart. According to one study: "This investigation indicates that candidiasis occurs when the host's environment is altered, primarily by antibiotic therapy. Candida then can colonize lining surfaces, and from there invade adjacent vessels and disseminate throughout the body."[1]

The most obvious stressor that can trigger yeast overgrowth is the presence of refined or concentrated carbohydrates, especially in the form of sugars. High levels of carbohydrates are especially problematic when combined with high levels of fat in the diet because fats tend to inhibit our cells' ability to absorb blood glucose, as described in the previous chapter.

Other factors that can contribute to yeast overgrowth include antibiotics, hormonal problems, birth control pills, alcoholic beverages. and emotional stress.[2] Some health care practitioners also believe that toxic metals such as mercury fillings can contribute to yeast overgrowth.[3]

> "Antibiotics can predispose the human body to systemic yeast overgrowth."[4]

## Foods that Feed Fungus

Nutritional authors have varying views on how to eliminate candida over growth. However, there is general agreement that the following should be restricted or avoided:
- White bread
- White rice
- Cookies, cakes, and candies
- Processed and smoked meats
- Dried fruits
- Fruit juices
- Leftovers
- Any preserved food, such as pickles, that is likely to have yeast or other fungi.
- Fresh fruit may or may not be restricted, depending on the dietary strategy you choose, as described below.

## Foods to Include

- Generous helpings of vegetables.
- Wild-caught fish, pasture raised meat, free-range eggs.
- Nuts and seeds, preferably raw. Get them fresh and keep them refrigerated so as to minimize oxidation of the fats and growth of fungus.
- Whole Grains – especially brown rice, spelt, oats, and kamute.
- Pseudo grains – buckwheat, millet, and amaranth.
- Fruit in varying amounts, depending on the dietary strategy that is used.

### Fat-Based or Carb-Based Diet

The fat-based or carb-based plans for diabetes, described in the previous chapter, would also apply for resolving candida issues. In most systems, fruit is restricted. However, those who use fruits freely claim that fruit is not a problem, provided that the fruit is fresh and the fat intake is low.

In addition to using one of the above plans, some individuals do a so-called candida cleanse. There are a number of ways of doing this, but the essential features are antifungal agents and probiotics.

## Anti-Fungal Agents

Anti-fungal agents are used to kill yeast and other fungi. Non-prescription topical pharmaceutical products are available, as well as powerful prescription drugs for internal use. In addition, many herbal and food-based products are available. For example:
- pau d'arco
- caprylic acid
- oregano oil
- citrus seed extract
- grape seed extract
- cloves oil
- garlic
- ginger
- aloe vera

## Probiotics

One of the vital functions of our beneficial bacteria is to inhibit the overgrowth of potentially harmful organisms such as candida. These bacteria are found abundantly in the small and large intestines. The best-known are acidophilus and bifidophilus. Beneficial bacteria are also found in the mouth, throat, air passages, skin, and the urinogenital tract of both males and females.

Women who take antibiotics often experience a vaginal yeast infection because the drug decimates the beneficial bacteria which normally produce lactic acid that inhibits the proliferation of yeast. However, the unconformable yeast overgrowth on the vaginal wall is just the most obvious manifestation of a more widespread problem that occurs in both males and females who take antibiotics.

Probiotics supplements, as described in Chapter 5, provide a relatively quick and convenient way to infuse the gastrointestinal tract with beneficial bacteria. For vaginal hygiene, a probiotic or lactic acid douche may be used. This can be a great blessing after taking antibiotics.

**Fermented Foods**

An alternative to probiotics is the use of high-quality fermented foods which contain live cultures of beneficial bacteria and their byproducts. However, some fermented foods, such as kombucha, contain yeast, and should therefore be avoided. In fact, some practitioners would eliminate fermented foods altogether from the anti-candida diet because of the possibility of harboring yeast and other fungi. Nonetheless, the right kind of fermented foods can be made in ways that exclude yeast and fungal infestation. Such foods include yogurt made from dairy milk or coconut, sauerkraut, kimchi, and various other forms of cultured vegetables.

High quality fermented foods provide a number of benefits besides helping to correct yeast overgrowth. Fermentation tends to increase the nutritional value of the food, as well as making it easier to digest. Fermentation produces B vitamins, omega-3 fats, glutathione, enzymes, lactic acid, and various substances that benefit the immune system, reduce allergic reactions and lower inflammation. Fermentation also improves the absorption of nutrients into the blood, most notably minerals. Lactic acid in fermented foods promotes intestinal motility and inhibits the growth of potentially harmful organisms, such as salmonella, E coli, ameba, and worms.

The use of probiotics and/or fermented foods is especially beneficial after the individual takes the above-mentioned antifungal agents because they often decrease the population of beneficial bacteria, along with the yeast.

To assure that you are getting substantial therapeutic value from these products, get the highest quality you can. The best probiotic supplements tend to be more expensive; they are often refrigerated and frequently found in glass containers.

High quality fermented foods are also available in some health stores and supermarket. However, the best fermented foods are typically homemade, as described on the next page.

# How to Make Cultured Vegetables

For best results, make cultured vegetables at home, using organically or naturally grown ingredients, and consume them at the height of freshness and nutritional value. Below are guidelines for making cultured vegetables.

1. Start with one to three pounds of any combination of the following: cabbage, boc choy, cauliflower, broccoli, beets, carrots, cucumbers, zucchini, daikon radish, kale, Brussels sprouts, collards.
2. About one teaspoon of salt per pound of vegetables (optional)
3. One teaspoon of caraway seeds per pound of vegetables (optional)
4. Half a clove of garlic per pound of vegetables (optional)
5. Finely shred the leafy vegetables and cut the coarse vegetables into small pieces or thin slices.
6. Pound the vegetables for five to ten minutes to bring out the juices.
7. Infuse the mixture with starter culture of beneficial bacteria. This will promote the rapid growth of a thriving population of bacteria, which will, in turn, discourage the growth of yeast and fungus in the ferment.
8. Pack the vegetables into mason jars or crock pot. Keep the lids loose, so the fermenting vegetables can release gases.
9. Store at 68-75 degrees F$^o$ for three to seven days, then refrigerate.
10. Fermentation time depends on room temperature and how much salt is used. Lower temperatures and higher salt content translate into slower fermentation. Likewise, higher temperature and lower salt content translates into faster fermentation, but greater likelihood of mold.

# Chapter 17
# Safe and Effective Weight Loss

The Signal
The Foundation for health Weight Loss
Mother Nature Has the Answer
Two Dietary Strategies
Guidelines for Losing Weight

I once gave a presentation on healthy eating to a group of employees in large corporate office. The following year, I gave another presentation in the same location. One employee who had attended my previous talk came up to me and said that she had applied the information I shared the year before. She happily reported that she lost 35 pounds over a period of about six months. She also said that the process was fun and easy. She felt great and the weight stayed off. What did she do to get such great results with ease and grace? She basically applied the principles described in this chapter.

Obesity has reached epidemic proportions in industrialized nations. This is serious because obesity is not just an aesthetic problem. There is a greater likelihood of developing just about any health problem as body-weight increases beyond the ideal range. For example, as body fat increases, inflammation can happen more easily, which, in turn contributes to cardiovascular disease, cancer, and other degenerative diseases.

For most individuals, letting go of extra pounds is actually very simple. Unwanted weight gain is the result of ingesting more calories than we burn on any given day. However, simple is not the same as easy, as many individuals have discovered. There are certain elements of modern life that make weight gain very easy and weight loss difficult. The specific reasons are described below, but essentially, they may be summarized as a failure to receive the "signal."

# The Signal

Eating lots of calorically dense food is the most obvious reason for unwanted weight gain. The other reason is lack of exercise. The human body is not designed to be sedentary. Therefore, weight loss programs guide the individual to eat fewer calories and exercise more. The rest is details. In other words, the basic strategy for healthy weight loss is to eat less and exercise more.

So, why do many individuals find this simple strategy difficult to implement? A major reason is a numbing of our natural eating instincts. The same instincts that tell us what to eat and when to eat should also tell us when to stop eating. The stop signal (satiation) is activated in response to three primary factors:

- The presence of bulk in the stomach. As the stomach becomes fuller, we feel less inclined to eat.
- The presence of sufficient calories. The more calorically dense the food, the more quickly we feel satiated.
- The presence of sufficient micronutrients in the food, especially minerals.

There are other known and probably unknown nutritional factors that tell the brain when it is time to stop eating. There are also nonfood factors that influence how much food we eat and how easily fat get stored. For example, hormonal imbalances can influence how many calories a person consumes, as well as the proportion of calories which are burned or stored as fat. Likewise, extra body fat can *cause* unbalanced hormones — which means that the two (extra body fat and hormonal imbalance) can form a vicious cycle wherein each side amplifies the other.

Emotional factors must be considered in order for any diet to work. Indeed, emotions are often the reason that a particular diet doesn't work. The emotional factors are often linked to a lifetime of experience, during which food and eating habits gradually and insidiously become woven into the individual's daily pattern of things to do to feel "normal" in the presence of various stressors. In other words, the individual develops a food addiction.

When we factor in emotions and hormones, we can understand why losing extra weight is not often not easy. Nonetheless, the foundation for healthy weight loss is to work with the three core factors that control satiation, described above.

# The Foundation for Healthy Weight Loss

All three satiation factors must be fulfilled in order for the nervous system to tell us when to stop eating. More specifically, our meal should have enough calories, bulk, and micronutrients to allow us to feel satisfied and reduce body weight, while still meeting all other nutritional needs.

Fulfillment of these three requirements is easy when meals include generous amounts of food that is close to the way Mother Nature presents them. The less we process food, the more clearly our instincts can guide us.

As foods become more processed, the three satiation factors become progressively unbalanced. Processed food has less fiber (less bulk), less micronutrients, and more calories. This is the primary reason that so many folks become overweight and undernourished.

To understand how to apply the above information to facilitate healthy weight-loss, let us first consider how the body stores fat. Calories come from carbohydrates, fat, and protein. All extra calories, regardless of their source, can theoretically be stored as fat. However, there is a difference in the manner in which the body metabolizes carbohydrates, fats, and protein. The body tends to burn carbohydrates first and fats second. Protein is a distant third, because the body prefers to use it as a building material for making skin, muscle, bones, and other tissues, rather than burning it as fuel.

If the individual consumes more calories than needed on any given day, the body will preferentially burn the ingested carbohydrates, while storing the fat. Why does the body burn carbohydrates before fat? Quite simply, carbohydrates are easier to burn. The body can burn huge amounts of carbs quickly, efficiently, and cleanly. However, the body can store only a limited amount carbohydrate. The situation with ingested fat is reversed: fat burns slowly but can be stored very easily – in substantial amounts!

As two sources of energy, carbohydrates and fats are perfectly matched! They complement each other to meet all of the body's energy requirements. Carbohydrates provide the fast-burning fuel for situations that require large amounts of energy for immediate use. In contrast, fats provide slow-burning fuel for sustained long-term use.

Fat is also the ideal way to store surplus fuel because it packs the maximum calories into the minimum amount of space. In addition, ingested fat can be quickly stored without major alterations or energy expenditure. On the other hand, the body must expend energy to convert extra carbohydrates into body fat. Therefore, the body will do so only if it has more carbohydrates than it can burn at any given time.

## Mother Nature Has the Answer

There is a conspicuous absence of obesity among wild animals and pre-industrialized human societies living on whole foods. Likewise, our prehistoric ancestors living in the wild were unlikely to become obese because they simply did not have the luxury of being able to over-consume calories. On the contrary, their main challenge was to get enough calories to keep from starving. The situation is reversed for modern humans living in industrialized areas where calories are plentiful. More, specifically, there are three main features of modern diets that promote obesity:

- Unlike our ancestors, we have an abundance of high-calorie foods in the form of grains, starchy vegetables, dry legumes, nuts, seeds, and animal products.
- These same high-calorie foods are relatively low in bulk and micronutrients, resulting in a delay of satiation. This is especially true for highly processed foods — white flour, sugar, and extracted oils such as vegetable oils, coconut oil and butter. To complicate matters, many processed have been formulated to maximize consumption. Therefore, by the time the stomach feels full enough to give us a good clear stop signal, we have already over consumed calories.
- Eating too many calories is especially easy when a given meal is laden with both carbohydrates and fats. Any given whole food provided by nature typically has carbohydrates or fats as the major source of calories – if one is high, the other is low. For example, whole grains and legumes provide the bulk of calories from carbohydrates, while having modest amounts of protein and fat. Nuts and seeds provide the bulk of calories from fat, with smaller amounts of protein and carbohydrates. Animal products typically provide their calories from fat and protein, with little or no carbohydrates.

In contrast, the mixing of high-carb and high-fat foods is quite common in our culinary creations: pizza, sandwiches, meat and potatoes, spaghetti, and tomato sauce (typically made with generous amounts of olive oil), cookies, cakes, and candies. With such foods, we can easily max out on calories.

# Two Dietary Strategies for Weight Loss

## The Low-Carb Strategy

Low-carb diets typically provide the bulk of calories from fat, while reducing carbohydrates. In addition, some of these diets often include higher levels of protein. One reason that weight loss occurs quickly with low-carb diets is that the digestion and metabolism of protein and fat takes longer and requires the body to expend more energy (burn more calories), compared to the digestion and metabolism of carbohydrates.

In other words, the body burns fuel less efficiently when it has to rely on very high levels of fat and protein. Burning protein for energy is inherently inefficient. Fats can burn efficiently, but to induce rapid weight loss, the diet is frequently adjusted so it becomes ketogenic, which essentially means that some of the fat-calories will not be burned but excreted.

The problem with burning fuel inefficiently is that it often results in toxic by-products. The rapid burning of fats produces ketone bodies, which are toxic if allowed to accumulate. The burning of protein results in the production of ammonia and other toxic substances. Long-term exposure to the elevated levels of toxins translates into accelerated aging and degeneration. Therefore, individuals who choose the low-carb approach for weight loss are advised to make sure that the diet has enough carbohydrates to prevent the excessive burning of protein and fat.

## The Low-Fat Strategy

The low-fat approach can be just as effective in weight loss, though it might take longer than high-fat-and-protein diets. The individual must simply reduce the high-calorie grains and starchy vegetables, while increasing fruits and low-starch vegetables. An example of such a diet is the one recommended by Dr. Joel Fuhrman. On his plan, even though total calories are reduced, the individual can still feel satisfied because the other two signals of satiation (fiber and micronutrients) are abundant. For the same reason, this sort of diet has been associated with cardiovascular health, strong bones, limber joints, cancer prevention, and reversal of diabetes.

Raw vegetables are especially effective for weight loss because they are rich in fiber and micronutrients, while having the least number of calories of all the food groups. In fact, some raw vegetables actually cause the body to burn more calories than the food provides! In other words, the more vegetables you eat, the more rapidly you lose weight – healthfully.

# Seven Guidelines for Losing Weight

Whether you favor the low-carb or low-fat approach, losing weight safely and effectively becomes very doable when you observe the following guidelines.

**1. Burn more calories than you consume.** This is the primary requirement. The remaining principles below provide the specific means for safely implementing this one.

**2. Make room for fresh fruits and vegetables.** Though calories are reduced, the diet should still provide an ample number of vitamins, minerals, and other nutrients. This is done by consuming enough fresh fruits and low-starch vegetables. As an added benefit, the increase in fruits and vegetables provides enough bulk to create a sense of fullness and satisfaction, even though calories have been reduced.

**3. Reduce high-calorie foods.** These foods are consumed in portions that are small enough to allow for healthy weight loss, while providing sufficient calories and nutrients to run the body. High-calorie foods can include clean sources of protein, fats and carbohydrates, such as grass-fed beef, free-range poultry, wild caught fish, eggs, beans, whole grains, and starchy vegetables (potatoes and winter squash).

**4. Avoid mixing high-fat and high-carb foods.** One of the main causes of unwanted weight-gain is eating meals that have both large amounts of carbohydrates and fats. We can avoid such combinations by reducing either the carbohydrates or fats in the same meal. For example, if your meal has a substantial amount of meat or cheese, you would avoid large amounts of high-starch foods, such as potatoes or bread, or use them sparingly in that same meal. If your meal has large amounts of high-carb foods such as pasta or rice, you would avoid animal products and other fatty foods, or use them sparingly. By not mixing large amounts high-carb and high-fat foods, our natural stop signal tends to work better. *All major dietary systems do this to some degree.*

> By not mixing large amounts high-carb and high-fat foods, it is much easier to avoid over-consuming calories.

### 5. Eat Simply

The more we process and mix foods, the harder it is to avoid over-consuming calories. If a meal consists of simple combinations which are naturally tasty and satisfying without a lot of strong spices, the body can more easily sense when it has had enough food. For example, tender vegetables such as romaine lettuce and baby spinach can be used to create simple salads that are surprisingly tasty and satisfying. High-quality fruit is typically tasty with no processing or cooking at all. Furthermore, even though fruits tend to be relatively low in calories, they still have enough to allow us to reduce our intake of calorically dense foods which are easy to overcome. In fact, a given type of fruit might be tasty and satisfying enough to be a meal in and of itself. Or, fruit can be the first course of meal. The second course can be a salad or a simple vegetable and meat dish.

### 6. Exercise

Exercise burns calories. More exercise burns more calories. In addition, exercise helps regulate appetite. Regular exercise also promotes emotional stability, thus reducing the need for "comfort food."

### 7. Listen to Your Body

Both the low-carb and low-fat methods have been used safely and effectively to produce weight loss. It is just a matter of determining which is better for you.

# Chapter 18
# Hormonal &
# Reproductive Health

Metabolism
Reproductive Health
Hormones and Stress
The Food Connection
Tips for Regulating Hormones

Unwanted weight gain, depression, blood sugar issues, osteoporosis, breast cancer, menstrual difficulties, infertility, prostate problems, erectile dysfunction, and just about every health issue mentioned in this book, can be caused or aggravated by hormonal imbalances.

Hormone health is all about balance. To understand balanced hormones and how food plays a role in it, we will first consider a word that is frequently used in nutritional circles, but often not clearly understood — metabolism.

## Metabolism

Metabolism is the sum of all chemical reactions in the body.

Chemical reactions generally fall into two categories: anabolism and catabolism. Anabolism is the building of molecules, and catabolism is the breaking down of molecules.

A major function of our hormones is to regulate metabolism. Some hormones are obviously anabolic, others are catabolic. For example, testosterone triggers the building of muscle protein, while thyroxin causes our cells to break down or burn carbohydrates and fats for energy.

Individuals who burn fuel quickly are often said to have a "fast metabolism," which actually means that they have fast catabolism. Likewise, individuals who gain weight easily or have a hard time losing weight are often said to have a "slow metabolism," which means their capacity to catabolize or burn fuel is on the slow side.

| Glands | Hormones | Functions |
| --- | --- | --- |
| Pineal gland | Melatonin | Relaxation, sleep |
| Pituitary gland | Growth hormone | Protein synthesis for regeneration |
| Thyroid gland | Thyroxin | Burning of carbohydrates and fats to generate energy |
| Thymus gland | Thymosin | Maturation of T-cells for immune system |
| Adrenal glands | Adrenalin Cortisol | Prepare the body to handle stress |
| Pancreas | Insulin | Lowers blood sugar |
| Ovaries or testes | Testosterone estrogen progesterone | Maintain integrity of tissues, especially male and female characteristics |

Some hormones may trigger both anabolism and catabolism. For example, growth hormone, produced by the pituitary gland, triggers the building of proteins (anabolism). One such protein is collagen which is needed for making skin, muscles, bones, tendons and ligaments and the blood vessels. Growth hormone also triggers the burning of fat (catabolism), thus generating the extra energy needed to build collagen.

In addition to their direct effect on anabolism and catabolism, hormones have other effects, such as regulating blood sugar, cholesterol, body temperature, pH, and blood pressure. Hormones are also critically important for the male and female reproductive systems.

# Reproductive Health

To understand the common health challenges associated with the male and female reproductive systems, let us consider two points about these systems and their associated hormones:

- Estrogen and testosterone are considered sex hormones but have other important functions as well. They are both important anabolic hormones that do more than just maintain the sex organs. Testosterone promotes muscular development, while estrogen promotes bone and brain development. Both hormones are found in males and female. Both hormones have a profound effect on behavior. Testosterone is associated with assertiveness, competitiveness, and sexual behavior — in both males and females, while estrogen promotes positive mood. High testosterone can produce hostility, aggression, and suspicion, while high estrogen can produce mood swings. Low levels of both can cause depression, apathy, and cognitive decline

- The reproductive system in both sexes differs from other systems in that it is not primarily designed to support survival of the individual, but rather of the species. In that regard, the health of the individual is important during the reproductive years but not as much afterward. In the natural world, we see animals, such as salmon, which undergo rapid decline and death immediately after they reproduce. We see a similar post-reproductive degeneration in other animals, though less extreme in species, such humans, that care for their young. In fact, humans, as with other big-brained mammals, do not merely take care of the physical needs of the young, but also *teach* the young. Therefore, longevity clearly offers an adaptive advantage because the young can learn from the parent as well as the grandparents. Nonetheless, humans still experience post reproductive decline, though not as pronounced as many other animals.

**Hormones and Goldie-Locks**

The point here is that declining estrogen and testosterone levels after the reproductive years do not just affect the sexual organs and sexual behavior. They have wide-ranging effects. Even during the reproductive years, estrogen and testosterone can still become unbalanced by the stresses of daily living — including dietary stress. Throughout life, our so-called sex hormones must be maintained within an ideal "Goldilocks" zone — not too much and not too little.

Furthermore, when a given hormone is "balanced," this does merely refer to how much of it is actually in the body. Hormones must also be balanced *relative* to each other. For example, the overall physiological and psychological effect of a given amount of estrogen depends on how much testosterone and progesterone are in the body.

Seems like a complex balancing act. And it is. Keeping Goldie-Locks happy is often not as simple as giving her hormones. In fact, experience has shown us that hormone-replacement therapy should be done with great caution, because it can do more harm than good — even with the so-called bioidentical hormones.

Fortunately, we do have safe and natural methods that simplify the process of bringing balance to our hormones. A common cause of many hormonal problems is stress. Therefore, rather than tinkering with individual hormones, we can support the body in achieving hormonal balance by doing positive things to undo the physiological effects of stress.

## Hormones and Stress

As described in Chapter 9, when the body is sufficiently stressed, it "forgets" how to restore and rebalance itself. This is largely due to high levels of stress hormones and low levels of hormones associated with rest and regeneration. And that is just the beginning. Here is a more complete list of how stress throws hormones out of balance:

- Chronically high cortisol levels can contribute to insulin resistance, which leads to type 2 diabetes.
- Chronically high cortisol levels can disrupt the functioning of the thyroid gland.
- High levels of stress hormones during the day can inhibit secretion of melatonin at night, resulting in disturbed sleep. The next day, the person has low energy, and might rely on stimulants, such as caffeine, which further unbalance the endocrine system.
- High levels of stress hormones and low levels of melatonin result in the individual having a harder time reaching the deep dreamless sleep, during which the pituitary gland normally sends out its biggest surge of growth hormone. As expected, low levels of growth hormones result in inhibition of tissue regeneration.

In other words, stress triggers hormonal imbalance, which in turn, will stress the body further. The individual, literally, cannot relax and is trapped in a vicious cycle, in which the body ages and degenerates at an ever-increasing rate, as described in chapter 9.

The hormonal effects described above may be produced by any form of stress. One such stressor is food. Likewise, food may be used to help the body restore hormonal balance.

## The Food Connection

Certain foods or combinations of foods result in secretion of stress hormones, most notably cortisol, as described in Chapter 9.

Besides not overeating, there are two general guidelines for using food to positively influence hormones:
- Boost your ingestion of fresh produce.
- Eat within your zone

## Boost Fresh Produce Intake

The connection between fresh produce and hormones is less obvious than its connection with the digestive system, but equally profound. This becomes clear when we remember the obvious fact that the function of hormones is to regulate the physiology of the body. The nutrients found in food, as you may recall from Chapter 2, are used in three basic ways:
- Nutrients are burned as fuel
- Nutrients are used as building material
- Nutrients are used as agents of *regulation*

Modern diets have no shortage of fuel or building material — carbohydrates, fats, and protein. In other words, modern diets tend to have no shortage of calories. However, there is frequently a shortage of vitamins, minerals, and phytonutrients; these nutrients are all about regulation — just like hormones!

We need the regulatory power of vitamins, minerals, and phytonutrients. just as we need the regulatory power of hormones.

Now we can begin to understand how a nutritional deficiency can contribute to a hormonal problem. In one sense, lack of regulation from a nutritional deficiency puts a "strain" on the regulatory power of our hormones. For example, if we lack the vitamins, minerals and phytonutrients that normally promote insulin sensitivity, the pancreas has to secrete more insulin to compensate. Higher levels of insulin tend to make the cells even more resistant to insulin, thus necessitating even higher levels of insulin. A vicious cycle is established which eventually culminates in type 2 diabetes, as described in chapter 15.

There are many other examples of nutrients exerting their regulatory effects by influencing the levels or activity of hormones. For example, the mineral iodine is needed to make thyroid hormone. Zinc is needed by the pancreas to make insulin. Chromium helps insulin to bind to our body cells.

Some phytonutrients have been shown to favorably effect estrogen levels.[1] Quercetin, a common phytonutrient found in fruits and vegetables, can raise serotonin levels in the brain, which in turn can upregulate the production of the hormone, melatonin.

Both serotonin and melatonin promote relaxation and positive mood. In addition, melatonin can downregulate the secretion of stress hormones. In other words, through a cascade of physiological events, quercetin can help reduce the levels of stress hormones in the body.

### Eat Within Your Zone

As described above, increasing fruits and vegetables might be the simplest and perhaps most effective way to adjust food intake to promote balanced hormones — at least for some individuals. If this approach does not produce the desired results, the next step is to eat within your zone, which means that you adjust the proportion of carbohydrates, fats, and protein in your diet to allow for optimal utilization of all three.

By eating within your zone, you tend to create internal conditions wherein the body isn't compelled to pump out extra hormones to keep thing balanced. For example, the pancreas does not have to secret extra insulin to prevent spiking of blood sugar. The adrenal glands don't have to secret extra stress hormones to smooth out the physiological bumps created by the clash of carbs, fats, and protein in the gut and in the blood.

Your ideal zone will probably be the carb-zone or the fat-zone, which means that you will be eating a carb-based (low-fat) diet, or a fat-based (low-carb) diet. If you feel you need help in doing this, you can consult with a nutritional counselor. Or look into any of the established dietary systems that make sense to you — all of them are carb-based or fat-based, even if they do not call attention to it.

---

## Tips for Regulating Hormones

**Eat within your zone** and include fresh produce.

**Exercise.** Hormones, such as insulin, cortisol and melatonin have been shown to normalize with exercise.[2]

**Support your local liver.** The liver breaks down hormones. Chapter 5 gives guidelines for supporting liver function, but the bottom line is this: eat leafy green vegetables, such as kale, broccoli, and dandelion. Carrots and beets are good.

**Female reproductive issues.** Supporting the liver might be the simplest way to help balance female hormones. Supplemental omega 3 oils can also help. The use of soy products remains

---

controversial for female issues. Some studies suggest that the right kind of soy products can be beneficial, while others say otherwise. Appendix B addresses this issue in more detail.

**Male reproductive issues.** Garlic, pumpkin seeds, watermelon and beets can be beneficial for the male reproductive system. Acai juice and goji berries can help with erectile dysfunction. Antioxidants are especially important for prostate health.[3] Saw palmetto can help with prostate issues.[4] Zinc and vitamin E may also help with reproductive health.

**Blood sugar hormones.** One of the simplest ways of helping regulate blood sugar is to eat within your zone. This is especially effective when combined with regular exercise.

**Stress Hormones.** Easy on stimulants! Extra vitamin C, B vitamins, and omega-3 oils, can also help.

**Thyroid hormone.** Iodine is essential for making thyroid hormone. Sea vegetation such as nori, wakame, kelp and dulce are good sources of iodine. If you take iodine in supplement form, be mindful of not taking too much; follow the recommended doses on the label.

**Pituitary and pineal hormones.** Growth hormone, made by the pituitary gland, is needed for tissue regeneration. Melatonin, made by the pineal gland, is needed for rest and sleep — which is also essential for regeneration. Both hormones can benefit from exercise and good nutrition. Exercise is best when done outdoors, because sunshine helps regulate melatonin by allowing the pineal gland to rest properly during daylight hours. On the nutritional side, some of the phytonutrients in fresh produce promote higher levels of melatonin, as described in the chapter that follows.

# Chapter 19
# Youthful Brain

A High-maintenance Organ
Neurotoxins
Nourishing the Brain
Sanity and Sanitation
The Brain-balancing Diet
Exercising the Brain

What does the brain need in order to realize its potential for health and longevity? The simple answer is that it needs nutrients and must be kept relatively free of toxicity. In that regard, it is no different from other organs. So, what makes it so special that it has earned two whole chapters in this book? First, the brain has to perform at high levels of intensity, consequently its energy requirements are enormous. Furthermore, the brain is particularly vulnerable to damage.

The brain's nutritional requirements must be precisely met if it is to function normally and remain healthy. If its requirements are not precisely met, the short-term consequence is reduced functionality — foggy thinking and mood swings. The long-term consequences are accelerated aging and degeneration.

In other words, the brain is a high-performance organ and price for this high level of performance is that the brain is also a high-maintenance organ.

## A High-Maintenance Organ

If we imagine the other body organs as a team of mules, the brain would be more like a thoroughbred racehorse. The other body organs are relatively steady, resilient, dependable, and adaptable; they easily adjust themselves to meet the challenges of the moment and they make the best use of whatever nutrients we give them. In contrast, the brain is temperamental, finicky, demanding, hot-natured, high-strung, and skittish.

Physically, the brain is very vulnerable. It is so soft and watery that if it were to rest unsupported on a hard surface, it would flatten like an egg yolk. To protect this most delicate of organs, Mother Nature encases it in bone. In addition, its surface is cushioned from the bone by three blankets of soft tissue, called the meninges, which also serve as a container for cerebrospinal fluid. In essence, the brain floats in its own personal pool, without which it could easily be damaged by a mild blow to the head.

## A Picky Eater

Most other tissues in the body burn both carbohydrates (typically glucose) and fat for energy. In contrast, brain cells burn little or no fat, relying primarily on glucose.[1] In fact, the amount of glucose burned by brain cells is enormous.

We have glucose as our blood sugar primarily to feed the brain because it has the highest energy requirements of any organ. Though it accounts for only 2% of the body weight, the brain burns about 30% of the total fuel used by the body.

Just as the brain's energy needs are very high, its requirements for cleansing and regulation are also great. It exhibits heightened sensitivity to excessive work and not enough rest. It must also have extra protection from oxidative stress and other forms of toxicity. Such protection is provided by an arsenal of antioxidants and the so-called blood-brain barrier.

# Neurotoxins

Since the brain is so chemically sensitive, scientists have a separate category for chemicals that are toxic to the brain. These so-called neurotoxins include caffeine, MSG, alcohol, mercury, aluminum, and fluoride. They are found in foods, drugs, vaccinations, water, and personal care products.

- **Caffeine** is an alkaloid found in a number of plants, such as the coffee bean, green tea, and cocoa. When ingested in modest amounts as part of a whole food matrix, it is relatively harmless and might even have benefits for some individuals. However, high levels of caffeine raise cortisol levels. Chronically high cortisol levels kill brain cells.

    How high is too high? That depends. The adverse effects of a given amount of caffeine depend on the source (natural or artificial) and the presence of other stressors that might also raise cortisol levels.

- **Alcohol** has an immediate adverse effect on brain function, due to irritation of brain cells. It also has long term effects: destruction of brain cells, cognitive impairment, confusion, and paralysis. The long-term effects are believed to be due to severe thiamine deficiency produced by the chronic overconsumption of alcohol.

- **MSG** is an excitotoxin, meaning that it overexcites brain cells to the point of killing them. It is widely used in Asian restaurants, fast food restaurants, and packaged foods.

- **Mercury**, even at very low levels, triggers breakdown of brain cells. Sources of mercury exposure include dental fillings, seafood, certain soaps, drugs, and vaccinations. The amount of mercury in each of these might be minimal, but it accumulates over time from multiple doses.

- **Aluminum** has been associated with Alzheimer's disease.[2] It is a potent neurotoxin which is difficult to expel and tends to accumulate in the brain. Exposure to aluminum comes from personal care products, such as anti-perspirants, as well as aluminum cans, cook-ware, aluminum foil and vaccines.[3]

  When acidic foods such as tomato sauce are cooked and then stored in aluminum containers, aluminum levels can become dangerously high, and cause illness. However, as with mercury, even if aluminum levels are too low to be noticed, which is usually the case, it can still insidiously accumulate due to long-term exposure from multiple sources.

- **Fluoride** is a neurotoxin that tends to accumulate in the pineal gland.[4] Two common sources of fluoride are municipal water and fluoridated toothpaste. The amounts are supposedly too small to cause harm. However, these are not the only two sources of fluoride; it is also found in pesticides and other products that find their way into the body.[5]

  Furthermore, fluoride is not the only neurotoxin to which the brain is exposed. The official "safe" levels of a given neurotoxin are generally based on studies on the chemical used in isolation and do not account for the cumulative effects of multiple neurotoxins.

# Nourishing the Brain

To clarify and simplify the brain's nutritional needs, let us begin by remembering that the brain, like the rest of the body, uses all nutrients in one of three ways:

- Fuel — burned for energy
- Building material — assembled into brain tissue
- Regulation — used to regulate brain physiology

## Sugars

Glucose is what brain cells normally burn as fuel to meet their enormous energy requirements. In addition, glucose, and other sugars such as mannose and galactose provide the essential building blocks for making the receptors on the surface of brain cells that allow them to communicate properly with each other and their immediate environment.

All starchy foods provide the body with glucose. Fruits and young vegetables provide pre-digested glucose and other simple sugars. In addition, many plants reputed to have healing and brain-balancing properties, such as aloe vera, goji berries, algae, and certain mushrooms, have higher levels of the other sugars and polysaccharides which are specifically used to build those important receptors that allow brain cells to communicate.

The ideal source of sugars is whole foods, such as fruits, vegetables, and whole grains. However, sugars derived from refined carbohydrates, such as white sugar and white flour, should be minimized or avoided because they can result in foggy thinking, mood swings, and loss of appetite control.[6]

## Amino Acids

Amino acids derived from ingested protein provide building material for making brain cells. In addition, certain amino acids, are needed to make neurotransmitters and hormones, especially those which allow us to feel relaxed, peaceful, and happy. For example, tryptophan is used to make serotonin, a neurotransmitter associated with positive mood and calmness. Likewise, serotonin is absorbed by the pineal gland and converted into melatonin, which also promotes calmness and relaxation, as well as allowing us to fall asleep and stay asleep. Low levels of serotonin are associated with depression, anxiety, and insomnia.

Getting enough amino acids is fairly easy; you simply have to ingest adequate protein. Meat offers the highest concentration of protein. Turkey is particularly rich in tryptophan. Bananas are also a good source of tryptophan; certainly not as high as turkey, but like all fruit, bananas provide their modest levels of amino acids in a form that is easily digested or predigested, therefore, they can be quickly absorbed, without requiring a large energy expenditure by the digestive system. The latter may seem like a minor point, but a clear and unburdened digestive system can go a long way in keeping the finicky brain happy, as explained later in this chapter.

## Fats

The brain is the fattiest organ in the body and therefore requires adequate levels of the right kinds of fat to maintain itself. However, to properly understand the brain's need for fat, we must bear in mind that brain cells typically do not burn fat for energy.

Granted, fat can serve as an indirect source of energy for the brain, as in the so-called ketogenic diets. As previously described, when other body cells burn fat very quickly, they produce fragments of unburned fat molecules, called ketone bodies, which can be burned later by brain cells.

In other words, ketone bodies are chunks of fat molecules which have been effectively "pre-chewed" by other body cells into a form that the brain cells can use. However, there is a limit to how much energy brain cells can safely get from ketone bodies.

For the brain, the main value of fats is in their use as a key building material and as agents of regulation. As building material, polyunsaturated fats, especially omega-3, are important because they provide the ideal fluidity for the cell membrane, which is critically important for proper transmission of signals by brain cells. These signals are the physiological basis for clear thinking, emotional serenity, memory, and creativity.

Cholesterol is another important building material for brain cells. It tends to solidify or stiffen membranes, and therefore provides a stabilizing counterpoint to the fluidity of the polyunsaturated fats. In fact, one of the functions of cholesterol in the blood, including LDL, is to serve as a building material for regenerating and maintaining all body cells, especially brain cells.

The liver normally makes cholesterol in liberal amounts, so we have plenty to meet the needs of the body, including the brain. Cholesterol lowering medication has been associated with depression and impaired tissue regeneration, which might be related to inadequate levels of cholesterol.[7,8] For similar reasons, some authors theorize that a totally vegan diet might result in cholesterol levels that are too low to support proper mood in certain individuals.

Regarding polyunsaturated fats, omega 3 and omega 6 fats are the most prominent. Both are needed by the brain, but omega 3 are the ones that are generally in short supply in the civilized diet, while omega 6 are often excessive.

Most of the omega 3 in the brain is in the form of DHA (decasohexanoic acid). In fact, the brain has the highest concentration of DHA of all body tissues. The body makes DHA from other forms of omega 3, but we can get it ready-made from certain foods, such as fish, eggs, and sea vegetation.

Lack of DHA has been associated with depression, impulsiveness, aggression, reduced intelligence, sleep problems, temper tantrums, alcoholism, schizophrenia, and manic depression.[9,10] One study showed that when women supplemented with DHA during pregnancy and lactation, children's IQ at 4 years of age was higher, compared to control groups.[11]

## Micronutrients

In general, the function of micronutrients (vitamins, minerals, and phytonutrients) is to allow the body to make good use of macronutrients (carbs, fats, and protein). For example, micronutrients protect the body from the potential toxicity resulting from the burning of macronutrients.

Phytonutrients, found abundantly in colorful fruits and vegetables, have many protective properties which are critically important for long-term brain health. For example, some phytonutrients promote production of glutathione, a powerful detoxifier and antioxidant, as described in Chapter 3. Other phytonutrients such as flavonoids promote higher levels of brain chemicals associated with calmness and cheerfulness, as well as helping tone down the stress hormones associated with aggression, depression and destruction of brain cells. Flavonoids are found abundantly in fruits and vegetables, as well as certain herbs that are known for their relaxing and mood-elevating effects, such as chamomile, peppermint, passionflower, and St. John's Wart.

The antioxidant activity of micronutrients is particularly important. As described previously, antioxidants neutralize free radicals — highly reactive molecules that can cause harmful oxidation. Burning fuel for energy produces a lot of free radicals, which can damage sensitive molecules such as fats.

We can fully appreciate the brain's great need for antioxidant protection when we remember that it burns a lot of fuel — which translates into a lot of oxidation! The brain is also very fatty — and the fat which is most abundant in the brain also happens to be the one that is most sensitive to free radical damage — DHA!

The close proximity of free radicals to highly sensitive fats translates into a potentially dangerous situation. It's like storing a large amount of gunpower next to a furnace! Not surprisingly, much of the brain degeneration associated with senile dementia seems to be linked to free radical damage.[12]

Besides the burning of fuel, another source of harmful oxidation is iron. Just as a high level of iron can trigger oxidation of cholesterol in the blood, it can also trigger oxidation of delicate brain fats. In some studies, subjects with the highest levels of iron showed the poorest cognitive performance.[13] This might explain why Alzheimer's disease has been associated with high iron levels and larger amounts of red meat in the diet.[14]

Bottom line, controlling oxidative stress is critically important for maintaining long-term health of the brain. The body responds to this great need by making powerful antioxidants such as superoxide dismutase and glutathione. In addition, we need the antioxidant power provided by some vitamins, minerals, and phytonutrients, found abundantly in fresh produce.

**Balance**

All of the above nutritional factors are needed for optimum brain health. If any are in short supply, the brain suffers. Unfortunately, we often try to compensate for the lack of one nutrient by ingesting higher levels of others. For example, a person might be depressed and irritable from lack of exercise, emotional stress and deficiency of vitamins, minerals, and phytonutrients, but tries to compensate by giving the brain extra carbohydrates, protein, or omega-3 oils, because these are easily accessible and often produce quick results. The downside is that such measures often produce short-term gain and long-term loss. Why? In general, there is likely to be long-term loss if we just try to get rid of symptoms, without addressing the problem at its source. For example, trying to fix depression or low energy by loading up on carbohydrates will probably do more harm than good, because it will overtax the body's ability to transport and metabolize sugars. In other words, don't give the brain extra fuel if there is no actual shortage of fuel in the first place!

The more typical way in which we try to balance brain function is by increasing protein or fat. Eating extra protein provides additional amino acids, which can help the brain up-regulate production of neurotransmitters. This is a more sensible approach than loading up on sugar but, here again, we should be cautious about relying on this method as a long-term cure. As a rule of thumb, the proper amount of protein to feed the brain should be the same amount that allows for proper nourishment of the body as a whole.

Granted, some depressed individuals feel better when they eat additional protein – even when the protein levels in the diet were already more than adequate. In such situations, it is quite possible that increased protein is compensating for some other hidden problem, such as lack of omega-3 oils — which is much more likely to happen than a true protein deficiency.

Taking extra omega-3 oils, usually in the form of fish oil, often have immediate, uplifting effects on mood and cognitive function. However, here again, we must be mindful of the long-term consequences of over-consuming protein or highly sensitive omega-3 oils. Giving the body extra protein means that the surplus will be burned as fuel, which creates long-term toxicity. Likewise, giving the body extra omega-3 can expose the body to added oxidative stress. Both of these low-grade stressors, can accelerate aging of the brain.

The fishy smell of an omega-3 supplement is a sign that it has already undergone substantial oxidation and is therefore toxic. The solution? Get your omega-3 from fresh whole foods whenever possible, and make sure that the increase in ingested omega-3 is matched by an equally generous increase in antioxidants.

As described in Chapter 2, whatever we do to fix an immediate health problem, it should not force us to pay for our short-term gain with long term loss. Balance is the key. Yes, supplements can be helpful in addressing an immediate health concern, as long as they are used judiciously as part of larger plan wherein the body gets the food, exercise, and rest needed to maintain health.

> Whatever we do to fix an immediate health problem, we should be mindful that we don't pay for short-term gain with long-term loss.

# Sanity and Sanitation

Yes, we can often experience an immediate psychological and physiological lift by taking additional amino acids and omega-3 fats. However, similar benefits have been noted when the body is simply allowed to gently cleanse itself more thoroughly than usual. Indeed, this could very well be the hidden underlying cause of the problem or at least one of the causes.

We are reminded here that good nutrition has two sides – a feeding side and a cleansing side. As with the rest the body, the brain needs to be kept free of waste products and other potentially harmful substances. A major source of such toxicity is the digestive tract.

## Poopy Thoughts

Mainstream medicine used to dismiss the idea that intestinal toxins can enter the blood and adversely affect brain function. However, this idea is now getting a fresh look, largely due to the awareness of leaky gut, as described in Chapter 5.

Essentially, leaky gut is a condition involving loss of integrity of the inner lining of the gastrointestinal tract, resulting in leaking of undigested protein, toxins, and intestinal microbes into the blood. This condition has been associated with cognitive decline and depression.[15]

One way of allowing the gut to cleanse and heal itself is by temporarily increasing the proportion of cleansing foods and decreasing the high-calorie building foods. Another way is to just give the GI tract some down time by fasting for a while. In addition, fasting is a time-honored method of inviting mental clarity and emotional steadiness. It is a common practice in many religious traditions. Fasting individuals often report insights, enhanced creativity, greater self-awareness, and clarity. On the emotional side, they report serenity and joyfulness. There is currently little data to explain the effects of fasting on consciousness, other than testimonials. However, according to one study, fasting animals show a reduction in the levels of certain enzymes called monoamine oxidases (MAO).[16]

The function of MAO is to help with detoxification. These molecules are normally found in high concentrations in the gut. They are also found in the brain where they promote breakdown of serotonin and other brain chemicals associated with calmness and happiness.

The above cited animal study offers a tantalizing model for explaining the connection between internal sanitation and sanity. Specifically, it is quite possible that the reduction of these enzymes during fasting allows for higher levels of the feel-good brain chemicals. It would be interesting indeed if a similar study was done with human subjects, so as to correlate their MAO levels with their subjective experience during a fast.

The point here is that sanitation in the gut correlates with the degree of mental clarity and emotional serenity. It is therefore not surprising that higher levels of fruits and vegetables in the diet have been associated with positive mood, as described below.

## Fruits and Vegetables

Fruits and vegetables tend to leave the least amount of toxic residue of the food groups which, theoretically, might allow for lower MAO levels. Furthermore, fruits and vegetables contain natural MAO inhibitors.[17] For example, one study suggests that a healthy diet can provide enough quercetin (found in commonly-used fruits and vegetables) to lower MAO and therefore modestly elevate the feel-good neurotransmitters in the brain.[18] These findings are consistent with other studies linking the consumption of fruits and vegetables with positive mood.[19]

# Brain-Balancing Diet

As with other health issues, we have two basic dietary options for healing the brain – a fat-based diet or a carb-based diet.

## Fat-Based Plan

Even before we delve into the specifics, the use of fat-based diets to support brain function seems logical, because the brain is the fattiest organ in the body! And indeed, in recent years, some exciting findings have emerged regarding the use of fat-based diets to address some neurological conditions, such as epilepsy, Alzheimer's disease, and Parkinson's disease. Individuals with these conditions often experience significant improvement when they go on a fat-based ketogenic diet. The challenge is to adjust the diet so that it is also sustainable for long-term maintenance. This usually means that carbohydrates are low, but not so low as to subject the body to high levels of ketone bodies or the prolonged toxicity of burning protein for energy. The other feature that makes the fat-based diet sustainable as a long-term maintenance diet is to include ample amounts of fresh produce.

### Carb-Based Plan

Carb-based diets have not been as closely examined as fat-based diets for supporting individuals with neurological problems. In fact, the success of fat-based diets in this area has been used by some dietary promoters to vilify carb-based diets in general. In essence, they claim that carbohydrates, especially glucose and fructose, are toxic and therefore should be consumed only in small amounts – by all humans! However, this assertion is based on clinical findings involving individuals suffering from neurological conditions, who may indeed be constitutionally compromised in their ability to process high-carb foods.

This is a good time to remember that a good therapeutic diet for a given subset of humans does not necessarily translate into a good long-term maintenance diet for everyone. If we wish to consider the possibility of applying any therapeutic diet as a long-term maintenance diet for *all humans*, we must first consider the bigger picture. In this case, we should consider the many studies done on traditional and modern populations eating carb-based diets that show good health and longevity – and a very low incidence of brain-related illnesses.[20]

This is also a good time to remember that good nutrition is about relationship. In this case, the manner in which carbohydrates behave in the body depend on what the rest of the diet is like. We should be cautious about pointing to one isolated nutrient as the cause or cure for an individual's health problems.

### Grain Brain?

One of the conclusions regarding people with neurological conditions, is that they may be unable to properly process grains, especially glutinous grains. However, this does not necessarily mean that *everyone* should eliminate *all* grains! Furthermore, there are other ways of eating a carb-based diet, besides relying heavily on grains. Legumes, potatoes, sweet potatoes, winter squash, fruits and vegetables are all carb-based foods.

Granted, fruits and low-starch vegetables are low in calories, but they can still make a significant caloric contribution. In fact, some vegetables, such as kale, collards, kohlrabi, dandelion, broccoli, and cauliflower provide a surprisingly large number of calories, if used liberally in the diet.

In other words, it is possible to have a carb-based diet that restricts or even excludes all grains and potatoes; relying instead on larger amounts of low-starch and semi-starchy vegetables, as well as fruit. Such a diet will be rich in vitamins and minerals, as well as providing a wealth of brain-benefitting phytonutrients.

**Common Features**

Whether you choose a fat-based or carb-based diet to support brain health, here are some guidelines that would apply to both:

- Favor foods that are **anti-inflammatory**, rich in **antioxidants** and rich in nutrients that promote **nitric oxide**. These foods are listed on pages 33-35.

- Load up on **Phytonutrients**. In addition to providing critically important antioxidant protection, phytonutrients provide regulatory support to help the brain maintain the proper levels of neurotransmitters. This is easier to do with a carb-based diet that features higher levels of fruits and vegetables. However, even a fat-based diet can include ample amounts of fresh fruits and vegetables because these foods are relatively low in calories while still providing a wealth of micronutrients.

- Include ample amounts of **Healthy fats**. This is obviously easier to do on a fat-based diet. However, a carb-based diet can still include enough high-quality fat-based foods to support proper brain function. Regardless of which diet you choose, one of the major points to consider here is to get the **proper balance of omega 3 and 6 oils.** Healthy fatty foods include raw nuts and seeds, avocados, coconuts, free range eggs, fermented dairy products such as yogurt, and wild-caught fatty fish, such as salmon. These same foods also provide the amino acids which serve as building blocks for making neurotransmitters.

- Eat **Walnuts.** Nuts and seeds are good brain food, but walnuts deserve special mention. In addition to having beneficial fats, walnuts promote production of serotonin and provide phytonutrients that protect the brain.[21]

- Eat **Mushrooms**. Edible mushrooms have been shown to benefit the brain and may even help individuals with Alzheimer's disease.[22] One such edible mushroom is **lion's mane mushroom**, which apparently contains neurotrophic factors that promote regeneration of brain tissue.[23] In fact, the results with lion's mane mushroom have been so impressive that it is now sold as a brain-boosting supplement.

- Keep the **digestive tract clean**. A brain-benefitting diet is going to closely resemble the gut healing diets described in chapter 5. The reason? Gut health can greatly impact what goes on between the ears, as described in the next chapter.

## Exercising the Brain

The same physical exercises that benefit the entire body also benefit the brain. In addition, we can also exercise the brain directly — by simply using it. This is how we can stimulate the growth of new brain tissue and improve its functioning. Engaging the brain in intellectually challenging activity increases the production of neurotransmitters and causes brain cells to branch out and develop new connections. This, in turn, prevents or delays the onset of degenerative brain diseases such as Alzheimer's and allows patients to make a more complete recovery from strokes.

Curiosity, creativity, problem solving, and learning new information and skills rejuvenate the brain. The rule of thumb for brain regeneration is to do something new and different. Use your mind and body in ways that you have never used them before. If you think you have two left feet, learn to dance, especially structured dancing that requires "learning steps." If you consider yourself to be mechanically challenged, fix, or build something. If you feel most comfortable with technical activities, try painting or poetry. If you feel more at home with art and poetry and can't seem to memorize things, take a class in botany or anatomy.

In other words, do something new and different. Do something that is outside your box. Do something that you find intriguing and perhaps a little scary or a bit beyond your comfort zone. And do it without criticism or harsh judgment. Do it as a child would do it. Do it just because you want to.

# Chapter 20
# Mental Clarity &
# Emotional Serenity

Hazards of Civilization
Your Brain on Flavonoids
Lifting Depression
Freedom from Addictions
Freedom from ADD and ADHD
Peace at the Dinner Table

The previous chapter provides guidelines for overall health and longevity of the brain. This chapter offers additional guidelines for using nutrition to help overcome some of the more common manifestations of an unbalanced brain.

Proper nutrition can certainly affect mental clarity and emotional serenity. However, the arrow of causality can also point the other way, meaning that the workings of the mind can have a powerful influence on the types of foods we eat and how well the body digests and utilizes them. For this reason, the two sides can easily become entangled in a vicious cycle — a loop of mutual re-enforcement, until the imbalance becomes noticeable — often as depression, addiction, ADD and ADHD.

The good news is that the two sides can also establish a loop of positive reinforcement wherein each side benefits the other. Indeed, this is precisely what usually needs to happen if we wish to restore mental clarity and emotional serenity. In other words, we need to give attention to both sides of the equation — the food we take in and the thoughts we put out.

Depression is probably the most common manifestation of an unbalanced brain. Addiction is a close second. Attention deficit disorder (ADD) and attention deficit and hyperactivity disorder (ADHD) also seem to be on the rise.

# Hazards of Civilization

The stresses of living in artificial environments and eating an unbalanced diet impact the mind as well as the body, even before the disturbance receives a medical diagnosis. ADD and ADHD are extreme examples of sympathetic dominance, wherein the body is unable to relax and renew, as described in Chapter 9. Children with ADD/ADHD remind us that sympathetic dominance has become more the rule than the exception. We have lost contact with our inner stillness.

Consequently, the body cannot realize its potential for health and longevity and the mind cannot quiet down sufficiently to know itself. On a more practical level, our attention span — our capacity to focus on a single task and follow it to completion — has plummeted.

A body that remains in overdrive too long eventually becomes fatigued and vulnerable to illness. Likewise, a mind that spins its wheels for too long will work inefficiently, wastes time and energy, and is likely to become depressed: it loses its capacity to care and to take joy in life. Deep depression is an erosion of the will to live. Addiction might be a desperate attempt to restore it, but typically has the opposite effect.

Research points to the existence of several neurophysiological links between depression and addiction.[1] The two are often seen together in the same person. Even when they aren't, if one is obviously present the other is probably close by, lurking in the shadows, perhaps trying to avoid detection.

Compared to the other common hazards of civilization, depression and addiction are less socially acceptable and more difficult to talk about. For example, personal issues with diabetes or arthritis are typically easier to discuss than addictions or depression. Issues with the mind are easier to conceal or hold in denial — until they are too problematic to keep hidden. When the individual does finally address the issue, healing can begin.

Compared to depression and addiction, ADD/ADHD tend be easier to talk about — and more difficult to conceal — but can still impede one's ability to function. As with depression and addiction, ADD/ADHD seems to be more common now than in the past, especially in children. In fact, much of the concern about ADD/ADHD is their increasing prevalence in children.

Some would argue that the seemingly increased prevalence of ADD/ADHD is due to more frequent diagnosis, perhaps motivated by the availability of drugs such as Ritalin to reduce symptoms. Whether or not this is true, the frequent use of such drugs in schools to control behavior of children is cause enough for concern. Beyond the harmful side effects of the drugs, we should seriously question the practice of routinely getting children accustomed to taking mood-altering drugs. A more rational strategy is to first seek to resolve the condition at its source. The same would apply to depression and addiction.

**Treat the Cause**

As described in Chapter 4, therapeutic measures are more likely to succeed and less likely to have harmful side effects if we seek to address the cause rather than just trying to get rid of symptoms. Granted, the cause is often difficult to discern, especially with conditions involving the mind. However, the good news is that we don't have to pinpoint the cause in order to get significant improvement of these conditions. What's more, the cause is often linked to stressors which are well within our ability to remove or affectively manage.

Depression and addictions have been linked to stress.[2,3] Both have a strong connection with food, as do ADD/ADHD. Naturally, there might also be genetic tendencies. However, as with the physical ailments described in previous chapters, genetic weaknesses involving the mind don't have to manifest, provided that nutrition and other factors are properly addressed. On the nutritional side, a very common but frequently overlooked contributor to disordered mental and emotional states is a lack of phytonutrients such as flavonoids in the diet,[4]

# Your Brain on Flavonoids

With the rise of civilization thousands of years ago, the diets of our ancestors underwent a radical change from one that was rich in fruits and vegetables to one that was dominated by grains and perhaps significant contributions from meat and dairy. They obviously survived, but survival is not the same as optimum health.

Because of the reduced consumption of fresh produce, the levels of phytonutrients in the diet plummeted. The previous chapter described how phytonutrients, especially flavonoids, help regulate the brain. For example, some flavonoids seem to promote higher levels of serotonin and melatonin, which are associated with positive mental and emotional states. They seem to be anticonvulsive, anti-depressant and mood-elevating. They reduce anxiety, calm the mind, and facilitate muscle relaxation. They might even be beneficial in Parkinson's disease.[5]

Flavonoids are largely responsible for the mental and emotional benefits associated with certain herbs, such as ginkgo biloba, chamomile, St. John's wort, and passionflower. Similar brain-active flavonoids are found in commonly available fruits and vegetables. Studies done on flavonoid-rich fruits and isolated flavonoids indicate that these phytonutrients have the potential to protect neurons against injury, improve memory and cognition, and might help to prevent strokes.[5]

Based on the above data, lack of phytonutrients might be a hidden contributing factor for the high incidence of depression in industrialized nations.

## Lifting Depression

- **Get your phytonutrients.** Fresh fruits and vegetables are the most common source. The individual may get additional brain-benefiting phytonutrients by enjoying an occasional cup of herbal tea made from chamomile, St. John's wort, passionflower, and gingko biloba. Stronger versions of these herbs may also be taken in supplement form.

- **Stabilize blood sugar.** Even for someone who is not vulnerable to depression, fluctuations in blood sugar can cause mood swings. Those with depression can use one the two diet plans to help stabilize blood sugar, as described in Chapter 15. You may use whichever dietary plan that seems more appropriate for your situation, but either way, avoid refined carbohydrates and trans fats, and favor whole foods.

- **Get your healthy fats.** As described in the previous chapter, the brain needs more fats than the rest of the body, because it is a very fatty organ. This point is especially important for those who favor a carb-based (low fat) diet. Such diets can still work well, provided the fat is not *too* low. Omega-3 fats are especially important for proper brain function. Supplementation with omega-3 oils, especially DHA and EPA, have been shown to lift depression.[6,7]

  Brain cells often convert fats into phospholipids prior to using them. Not surprisingly, many individuals with depression often respond well to supplementation with phospholipids.

Commonly used phospholipid supplements include phosphatidylcholine and phosphatidylserine, readily available in health food stores.

Another fat which is vital for the brain is cholesterol. Just as high cholesterol levels in the blood are a risk factor for cardiovascular disease, low cholesterol levels are not good for the brain either. Low blood cholesterol has been linked to depression.[8] This is important to know for individuals taking cholesterol lowering medication. In addition, some dietary authors assert that vegans might suffer from depression and other brain issues due to inadequate levels of cholesterol. This is theoretically possible, but since the liver normally makes all the cholesterol needed by the body, individuals with depression are more likely to be deficient in the other fats described above. Furthermore, the individual with depression might be deficient in other nutrients, besides fats, as described below.

- **Get your amino acids.** Dietary protein is digested into amino acids which are used mostly as building material for making muscle, skin, bone, and pretty much all body tissues. In addition, small amounts are used for making neurotransmitters that are critically important for brain function. For example, the neurotransmitter, serotonin, is made from the amino acid, tryptophan. Likewise, dopamine is made from phenylalanine.

Both serotonin and phenylaniline are considered "feel-good" neurotransmitters. Low levels of both have been associated with depressions and anxiety. This is why those with depression often feel better when they take **supplemental tryptophan**. For similar reasons, higher levels of dietary protein have been used to help people with depression.[9]

As a point of caution, excess protein might also *contribute* to depression. Therefore, one should not blindly load up on protein as a shot-gun approach for treating depression.

As described in the previous chapter, the levels of protein that provide optimum health for the body in general should also be optimal for the brain. How much protein does the body need? Realistically, the amount will vary from person to person, but most nutritional authorities agree that the average moderately active adult female needs about 50 grams of protein, and the average male needs about 60 grams. These levels are easily obtained from the typical vegan diet, or an omnivorous diet with modest amounts of animal products.

Again, most of the protein we eat is used as building material to make flesh and bones. The amount of protein needed to make neurotransmitters is actually quite small.

If an individual with depression seems to immediately feel better by eating high levels of protein, this does not necessarily mean the person had a true protein deficiency. More likely, the sudden increase in protein created a surge of amino acids in the blood that temporarily up-regulated production of feel-good neurotransmitters. This could very well compensate for other hidden problems, such as lack of exercise, or deficiency of phytonutrients, omega-3 oils, or vitamin D — all of which are far more likely to happen than a true protein deficiency.

Bottom line: get *adequate* protein to nourish the brain and the rest of the body. And then address other nutritional needs that might be contributing to the problem.

- **Get your vitamin D**. Lack of sunlight in the winter can result in low levels of vitamin D, which has been associated with depression. Individuals with depression often experience a lift when they take a vitamin D supplement.[10]
- **Get your sun light**. In addition to promoting production of vitamin D, sunlight is needed to regulate the pineal gland which makes melatonin. Not surprisingly, those who are deprived of adequate sunlight are more likely to become depressed or suicidal. This might be partially responsible for the high rate of depression and suicide close to the arctic circle.
- **Get your exercise**. For the brain to properly regulate itself and utilize nutrients, exercise is essential. Among its benefits, exercise increases serotonin, which, in turn, is absorbed by the pineal gland and converted into melatonin. Exercise also stimulates the release of endorphins and promotes sound sleep.

# Freedom from Addiction

Here are some common products that tend to be addictive:

- **Grains** and some other seeds – contain opioids.
- **Dairy protein** produces opiate-like substances when improperly digested — which is very common.
- **Caffeine** stimulates the adrenal glands and therefore has the potential to be addictive. Anything that stimulates the adrenal glands can be addictive.
- **Red meat** contains high levels of uric acid, which stimulate the adrenal glands in a manner similar to caffeine.
- **Cooked food** in general might produce a subtle stimulation the adrenal glands, as well as triggering an immune response.[11,12]
- **MSG,** used widely in restaurants, especially fast foods, over-stimulates and kills brain cells.
- **Many allergens** are addictive by virtue of the fact that they stimulate the adrenal glands.
- **Alcoholic beverages** have a numbing effect on brain cells, resulting in a reduction of physical pain and anxiety. In addition, such products are made from fermented plant foods which often contain allergens that produce a low-grade stimulation of the adrenal glands.

## Addiction and Stress

Beyond the adrenal connection, addiction thrives on stress.[13,14] This is why individuals in 12-step programs are advised to avoid extremes. They are told to avoid becoming too hungry, too tired, too lonely, too agitated, too *anything.*

Addictions are often not recognized as such but are concealed behind a veil of denial or rationalizations. Even if the addiction is recognized, it tends to assert itself anyway, overpowering the will and putting to shame our best intentions. When willpower tries to overcome the feelings (such as food cravings), the latter generally win. To complicate matters, the self-recrimination that often follows the fall from the wagon is yet another stressor that drives addiction! In that regard, many addictions are self-perpetuating.

Food addiction, like all addiction, thrives on harsh judgment.

If the above description gives you the impression that addiction is like a monster too powerful to defeat, take heart. The same guidelines already given to overcome depression can also help with addiction, though the results may not be as fast or dramatic. For example, exercise can have an almost immediate uplifting effect on depression. The same exercise can also help overcome addictions; it might just take longer. For additional support, here are two specific options for addiction recovery:

- **Amino acids.** L-tryptophan, L-phenylalanine and L-glutamine have been found beneficial with various addictions, including drugs and alcohol.[15]
- **Adrenal support.** Since the adrenal glands are often involved in food addictions, the procedures for nourishing the adrenal glands, as described in Chapter 9, can be most beneficial.

## Freedom from ADD and ADHD

The general guidelines previously given for depression are also applicable to individuals with ADD/ADHD or anyone who has a hard time focusing and relaxing. More specifically:

- **Omega-3** supplementation has been shown to be helpful for individuals with ADD/ADHD.
- **Avoid overconsuming omega-6 oils.** Vegetable oils, most nuts and seeds tend to high in omega-6.
- **Avoid refined sugar.** This includes most cookies, candies, and cakes. In addition, many other packaged foods have added sugar. Read the label.
- **Avoid trans fats.** Such foods include cookies, candies, cakes, margarine, white bread. Read the label.
- **Avoid artificial food coloring**. Studies supporting this idea do exist.[16] Furthermore, there is no shortage of antipodal evidence in the form of reports from parent and health care practitioners. Add to this the fact that artificial coloring does not add value to foods and are harmful to the liver and kidneys, and we are left with no justifiable reason to keep them in the diet.
- **Read a book.** Turn off the computer, put the cell phone away, and read a physical book for at least 30 minutes. You might notice that it has an entirely different effect on your mental and emotional state than the same amount of time on a computer.
- **Exercise.** In addition to promoting good circulation to nourish the brain, exercise helps balance hormones and the sympathetic and parasympathetic systems, which will likely help individuals with ADD/ADHD.

# Peace at the Dinner Table

It is not surprising that so many cultures have a tradition of blessing food and giving thanks at the start of a meal. It is not just a matter of spiritual cultivation. The more peaceful the mind, the more value the body can receive from food.

A peaceful mind translates into an active parasympathetic nervous system, which promotes good digestion and absorption. In addition, if we pay close attention, we might notice that the habit of giving thanks and blessing food at the start of a meal has an uplifting effect on other aspects of our lives. The effect might be extremely subtle and perhaps beyond our capacity to verbalize. However, if we could put it into words, we might say that the mind is operating from a place where it is able to perceive the bigger picture of our existence.

Seeing the bigger picture means we have a better sense of our priorities. We have a better sense of where and how to invest our time, energy, money. We have a better sense of where to put our attention and where to invest our emotions. Seeing the bigger picture provides a sense of freedom, wherein we don't sweat the small stuff, while also having a heightened capacity to delight in little things such as a quiet conversation with a friend, while eating a simple and tasty meal.

Depression and addiction are two common manifestations of a mind that has lost sight of the bigger picture. Such a mind tends to fixate on minutia and obsesses about small details. This translates into a constant, low-grade stress that puts the body into perpetual sympathetic dominance — which, in some individuals, gets labeled as ADD/ADHD. However, whether or not it gets diagnosed, it eventually depletes the body of energy and exhausts the mind's capacity to care. This is depression in the making. To complicate matters, the same hypervigilance of the nervous system that causes us to sweat the small stuff, also numbs our capacity to feel pleasure. In particular, we lose the capacity to find joy in little things and therefore require more and more stimulation to feel alive. This is addiction in the making.

All this inner drama tends to ease up as we cultivate the ability to put the moment-to-moment events of the day into perspective. There are many ways of cultivating the capacity to see the bigger picture. Blessing your food and giving thanks at the start of each meal is one of them.

# Chapter 21
# The Bigger Picture

The Miracle of Soil
The Real Food Pyramid
The Circle of Life
Be a Producer
Support Your Local Farmer
From Sacrifice to Synergy

*"Soil is miraculous. It is where the dead are brought back to life.[1]"*

The purpose of this final chapter is two-fold:
- Review key principles for using food as medicine.
- Integrate those principles into the bigger picture of healthy living.

The bigger picture has to do with relationship. Healthy eating is possible only when it is part of a bigger picture of healthy living, which includes our relationship with other humans and with the earth which provides our food. There is a deep interdependence between our inner world and outer world.

For example, even after reading the preceding 20 chapters, the connection between food and health cannot be fully understood or properly applied until we consider the obvious fact that the human body comes from the earth. As an organic farmer friend of mine put it: "The body doesn't just come from the soil; the body *is* soil." This visionary farmer saw the human body as a small droplet of earth which rises up like a whirlwind that dances briefly as living flesh and then returns to the earth.

Looking at it less poetically and more biologically, soil becomes food which contains the nutrients that become our muscles, bones, skin, and vital organs. Therefore, food is only as good as the soil on which it is grown. This fact, obvious though it may seem, has been grossly neglected. Nonetheless, it is critically important for anyone who seriously wants to use food as medicine.

| Food is only as good as the soil on which it is grown. |
| --- |

# The Miracle of Soil

It is easy to overlook something that doesn't immediately harm us. It is easy to forget that the power of food to help restore health is derived from the soil on which food grows. Indeed, poor food quality is a major reason that modern humans get sick in the first place. Health-conscious individuals are generally aware of this, but what they usually don't fully appreciate is that a major contributor to poor food quality is lack of minerals. The lack of minerals in food is primarily due to the stripping of minerals from soil by chemical farming.

> The value of food for maintaining and restoring health greatly depends on the quality of the food, especially the mineral content.

The good news is that we do not need to sap the life out of the soil and compromise the quality of food in order to produce enough for everyone — and to do so in a way that is economically feasible. We have the knowledge and the means to grow food that is clean, nourishing, and affordable, while providing a good income for growers and distributers. What's more, the power to make this happen, ultimately resides in the hands of the consumer.

I address this topic more deeply in my previous book, *What Should I Eat? Book 1*. In essence, the path becomes clear when we recognize the profound state of unity between our personal needs and that of the Earth and all life upon it. Such unity is not merely a philosophical ideology. It has been scientifically verified over and over again. Its direct impact on our physical health is reason enough to pay attention to it. In addition, awareness of the unity of all life affects us emotionally and socially; and touches into our spiritual sensibilities.

The centerpiece of the Catholic Mass is the death and resurrection of Jesus Christ, which is for the faithful a solemn and sometimes deeply evocative way of acknowledging that death is not the end of life, but rather the gateway to new birth. We are reminded that life itself simply goes on.

The miracle of death and rebirth is also happening moment by moment beneath our feet. The earth is the final resting place for all life forms; as well as being the great womb in which new life is born. If the earth could speak, it might say, "Behold, I make all things new again."

"Here in the thin earthy boundary between inanimate rock and the planet's green carpet, lifeless minerals are weathered from stone or decomposed from organic debris. Plants and microscopic animals eat these dead particles and recast them as living matter. In soil, matter crosses and re-crosses the boundary between living and dead...

"For years, scientists viewed soil mainly as an inert sand-like substance for holding plant roots, into which we poured fertilizers. But soil is alive...Think of soil as the base of a pyramid. Stacked upon this are plants, then insects, and finally animals, each dependent on the creatures below it. The greater the number and diversity of soil organisms – that is, the broader the pyramid's base – the larger and more diverse will be the flow of nutrients among them, as they release fertility stored in the soil.[2]

> We have the knowledge and the means to grow food that is clean, nourishing, and affordable, while providing a good income for growers and distributers.

## The Real Food Pyramid

The secret for growing an abundance of clean and nourishing food is to grow it in a way that allows the base of the pyramid to be as broad as possible. Contrary to this, conventional agriculture, with its use of chemical fertilizers, pesticides, and herbicides, has narrowed the base of the pyramid considerably.

The most obvious consequence of narrowing the pyramid is thinning top soil — from 30 inches in the American Midwest of the 1800s, to four inches today. And again, it is not just a matter of quantity but also of quality. The soil itself has been severely impoverished. The level of minerals, organic matter and living organisms in the soil are all essential for producing food that truly nourishes and heals.

Chemical herbicides, pesticides and fertilizers don't just add toxicity to food. These same chemicals kill the life within the soil. They do so slowly and invisibly. Likewise, they slowly and invisibly damage the life and health of animals (including humans) who eat the food that is grown on the soil – as well as having to breathe the air and drink the water that has been laced with the same chemicals.

As an example. glutathione is a hugely important molecule found in many fruits and vegetables and also made by our cells. It is essential for detoxification, maintaining health and recovering from illness, as described in Chapter 3. A key part of glutathione is the mineral sulfur — which ultimately comes from the soil.

Sulfur, along with other minerals, has been severely depleted from the soil by the use of chemical fertilizers. These fertilizers stimulate rapid growth of plants. However, they provoke equally rapid depletion of minerals and soil microorganisms. With each harvest of crops through conventional agriculture, the mineral content of soil decreases, making the farmer even more dependent on chemicals to make the plants grow and protect them from disease and insects — to which the plants become increasingly more vulnerable.

## The Circle of Life

To fully appreciate the message of the pyramid described above, and to begin to see how to restore it, we need to see it as more than a pyramid. The process by which the Earth provides food might be better visualized as a circle.

A circle has no beginning or end. This particular circle is formed by soil organisms which feed plants, which feed animals. And then, the plants and animals feed the soil organisms. All work together; transferring energy from one organism to another, like a great circular bucket-brigade.

For life to go on, the energy which cycles from soil organisms to plants to animals and back to soil organisms, must be allowed to do so in an unrestricted manner. The circle must be unbroken. Furthermore, the circle of life on Earth is part of a vastly larger cosmic circle in which the sun is the most obvious participant. When harmony exists among the organisms of the Earth, the sun is able to join the circle, adding more energy to the ecosystem. This is how life goes on, expanding, transforming, and evolving in

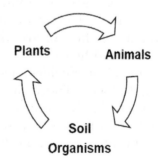

Plants    Animals

Soil
Organisms

accordance with Mother Nature's design.

On the other hand, if the circle of life on Earth is severely disrupted, the incoming energy from the sun cannot be born as new life. Instead, the same energy scorches the ground, turning it into a desert. Likewise, the rain that falls to the ground cannot nourish life either. It simply strips the soil of organic matter and usable minerals, leaving only sand and barren rock.

Since the entire system is cyclical, it makes no difference where the disharmony happens to be. If one part is neglected, the entire circle suffers. If the circle is broken anywhere, it is broken everywhere.[3]

## Broken Circle

Humans have now been practicing conventional chemical-based agriculture long enough to know that it produces short-term gain and long-term loss. This is the same mind-set that tries to fix immediate health problems in ways that produce future problems, as described in Chapter 4.

Conventional agriculture decimates soil organisms and depletes minerals. Conventional agriculture produces plants that might look good on the supermarket shelf, but are grossly deficient in nutrients and laced with poisons.[4,5] There is no shortage of studies showing that chemical residue from conventional farming is responsible for a number of emerging illnesses in modern humans, including a higher incidence of cancer and birth defects in those living on or close to conventional farms.[6] As described in Chapter 14, cancer is essentially a man-made disease, with chemical-based farming playing a major role.

On the ecological level, the number of animal and plant species that have already become extinct due to human intervention is so high that scientists have called it "the sixth great extinction," because it is on par with the five other mass extinctions which have occurred in the geologic periods of the past.[7]

## Mending the Circle

As suggested earlier in this chapter, we do possess the knowledge and the means to grow enough food for everyone and to do so in a way that maintains the quality of the food and integrity of the soil. Even now, such methods of food production are being studied and adapted to meet our current needs.[8]

Now the question is, what can we as consumers do about the manner in which food is produced? Besides being informed and letting the powers-that-be know that we are paying attention, there are two other things we can do, which are at least equally important to education and legislation:

- Be a producer
- Support your local farmer.

# Be a Producer

Growing your own food is a great hobby, offering a number of benefits on the personal, ecological, and social levels. If you take the time to learn how to maximize the quality of your soil, you will also maximize the quality of your food. What's more, since it comes from your own garden, it will be freshest and most nutritionally loaded that food you get. There is a huge difference between supermarket and freshly picked produce.

You can literally pick it eat it, which is how you maximize its overall nutritional value. If you avoid using all chemicals in your garden, the food you grow will be far cleaner and more nutritious than the typical produce from a store.

This is the sort of food which has the best potential for restoring life because it is fully charged with life. This is the sort of food that Hippocrates was talking about when he said, "Let food be your medicine, and medicine your food."

> The cleanest, freshest, most nutritious, and most health-giving foods are the ones you grow yourself.

There is even a theory that locally grown food offers protection from local pathogens. Plants do make chemicals that protect them from local viruses, bacteria, fungi, etc. When we eat these locally grown foods, we supposedly receive similar protection. Whether or not this is true, locally grown fruits and vegetables tend to be fresher, cleaner, and safer than produce that was grown thousands of miles away, because the latter has more time to pick up pathogens or become otherwise tainted while in transit or sitting in a warehouse.

At the very least, growing your own food is a great way to spend your free time, getting exercise, fresh air, and sunshine. It might also be one of the most potent and least expensive forms of psychotherapy. If done as a collaborative effort, as in a community garden, it is a great way for friends and family to gather. It is a place to have parties, share food, and nurture relationships in an easy and informal way.

Financially, if the garden is allowed to evolve properly, you will eventually save money. The savings will only increase as you become more knowledgeable about building soil and growing food. Over time, you will grow more food and better food, with less need for store-bought supplies. For example, by saving seeds, you will "breed" your own collection of seeds that are well-adapted to your soil and climate, and which do not have to be replaced by less-adapted store-bought seeds.

## Support Your Local Farmer

For most of us, growing all or most of our food is not practical. However, we can get virtually the same high-quality foods from small local farms. Neighborhood farmers' markets have become quite popular in small towns and large cities.

Just like the garden itself, the neighborhood farmer's market can offer other benefits, besides freshly picked food of the highest quality. Ostensibly, we go to the neighborhood farmer's market for the same reason we go to the supermarket. However, if we make a habit of it, we might find that it can nourish us in other ways as well. There is a certain satisfaction or reassurance that comes from buying food from the same person who grew it. The warm smile and look of pride as they describe how they grew the food seems to infuse it with more life-giving energy.

Like the garden itself, the neighborhood farmer's market offers other benefits besides freshly picked food of the highest quality.

There are other benefits as well. The neighborhood farmers market is a womb in which community is born. It is a gathering place where spontaneity and serendipity join hands in a simple and quiet way to bless both body and soul. It is fertile ground where friendship grows easily and organically in its own time and season.

"Farmers Markets are about more than food, more than farmers, more than 'buy local'. Farmers markets are about building communities and building relationships. They are about looking each other in the eye. They are about people more than product. Farmers markets help tear down barriers and build relationships. They give a community...heart.[9]"

In my other book, *What Should I Eat, book 1,* I describe how some health problems might appear to be food-related but really stem from emotional or spiritual issues which have been projected on food. For example, an individual might feel isolated or "empty" and attempts to fill the emptiness with food. This condition is pervasive in industrialized cultures. It is a brooding and gnawing hunger that can emerge in any social animal removed from its natural setting and isolated from others.

As with other primates, we humans are most assuredly social animals. Lack of friendship and the absence of community can produce a void that we may not be aware of, but unconsciously try to fill with food and other mood-altering substances. In that regard, the neighborhood farmer's market can be more than a market, just as the community garden is more than a place for growing food. Like fertile soil, it is a place where life touches life, thus creating new life.

## In Summary

The intellect may not be able to describe the precious element which makes life meaningful, but on the feeling level, it is plainly obvious. That feeling is our capacity to care. Without it, the information in the preceding chapters becomes futile because we drift into a state of mind which disrupts the working of the body and compromise its ability to be truly nourished by food.

In other words, effectively using food to recover from illness and optimize health is not merely about changing one's diet. It is about changing one's attitude toward food, especially an increased awareness of the source of the food.

The more we care about life, the more care about our health. The more we care about our health, the more we recognize the value of high-quality food. The more we recognize the value of high-quality food, the more we will be inclined to plant fruit trees, create vegetable gardens, and empower local growers who make it their business to grow clean and nutritious food.

# Appendix A
# The Egg Controversy

Some authors assert that eggs can be consumed freely. Others assert that eggs are unhealthy in any amount. To complicate matters, as with other food-related subjects, there is often emotional charge or vested interest around this issue. Consequently, the two sides often have difficulty communicating rationally to compare notes and learn from each other.

I personally have not consumed eggs in many years. However, prior to that, while living on a farm, I did eat eggs. I even went through a phase in which I ate eggs (more than one) just about every day for month. Coincidentally, I happened to check my blood cholesterol level during that time. It was normal.

To bring some clarity to this issue, let us first keep in mind that the egg controversy goes beyond cholesterol. We should also remind ourselves to use proper scientific caution and to free ourselves from the assumption that we already know all there is to know about this subject.

## What do we know?

Eggs have omega-3 oils, fat-soluble vitamins, high-quality protein and high levels of cholesterol and saturated fat, all perfectly blended to support the growth of a tiny chicken embryo into a fully formed chick, ready to hatch, in about three weeks. In other words, Mother Nature designed the egg to be a powerful building food — and herein lies the understanding of why eggs can be both useful and problematical.

## A Powerful Building Food

Building foods and cleansing foods are described in chapter 2. Essentially, building foods are those which are high in nutrients which provide the "brick and mortar" that make up the body, as well as the calories (energy) needed to assemble the nutrient molecules into living flesh. In that regard, eggs are, indeed, a powerhouse.

The main building materials making up the human body are protein and fat — both abundant in eggs. An egg is about 36% protein, 62% fat and 2% carbohydrates. The fat is mostly saturated fat, but also includes a decent amount of polyunsaturated fats in the form of omega-3 and omega 6. It is also very rich in cholesterol – another key building material.

Used judiciously, the building power of eggs can be helpful for those who need extra support in repair and regeneration, or who are recovering from the debilitating effects of a long-standing illness or chronic stress.

Using eggs judiciously means we remember that the nutritional needs of an adult human are different from that of a rapidly growing chick embryo. The latter thrives on a diet consisting entirely of the blend of nutrients found in the egg. Not so for humans, especially adult humans.

As described in chapter two, a major cause of disease in modern humans is too much of the building foods and not enough cleansing foods. More specifically, we tend to get too much protein, fat, and carbohydrates, and not enough vitamins, minerals, phytonutrients, fiber, and water.

A truly balanced diet is one that has the right balance of building foods and cleansing foods for a given individual. How do eggs fit into such a balanced diet?

### Different Yolks for Different Folks

Some studies link frequent egg consumption with cardiovascular disease, while others show no significant corilation.[1,2,3,4] As described in chapter 15, some studies link eggs to insulin résistance and type 2 diabetes. Other studies suggest that eggs might actually *improve* insulin sensitivity – for individuals who also limit carb intake.[5] However, moderation with eggs is still advisable for diabetics because they are apparently more likely to develop cardiovascular disease with increased egg consumption.[6]

When faced with such inconsistent or complex data, the rule of thumb is to use your common sense and personal life experience to guide your choices. Can *you* benefit from the added regenerative boost of high-quality farm-fresh eggs? Or are you one of those individuals who might be better off without eggs? And, if eggs *are* a healthy food for you, how many should you eat? In my opinion, *you* are ultimately the best judge of that.

If you do feel inclined to eat eggs, select the highest quality. The eggs in most stores come from factory-raised chickens which have been raised under extremely unsanitary conditions, are loaded with antibiotics, and are subject to salmonella. Eggs derived from properly fed free-range chickens are available in health food stores, some supermarkets.

The best eggs will have a yolk that is firm and deep orange in color. It will also be tastier than eggs that come from factory raised chicken. The highest quality eggs may be obtained from local farms, neighborhood farmer's markets or your own free-range chickens. Such eggs are so loaded with nutrients that we really don't have to eat that many to receive their health benefits.

# Appendix B
# Is Soy Good for You?

To properly answer the above question, we should first pay attention to its wording. The question asks whether soy is good for *you* — not *us*. In other words, my purpose here is to help you determine if soy would be beneficial for *you* personally, not for all humanity. I emphasize this point because there is much controversy about soy in the world of diets and nutrition. Some nutritional authors praise it, while others reject it. Both can be quite persuasive, backing up their assertions with scientific studies, leaving sincere health seekers scratching their heads.

Part of the issue is that much of the available data have been filtered through parties that have a vested interest in promoting soy or vilifying it. For example, some of the popular pro-soy literature is promoted by the multibillion-dollar soy industry or vegetarian authors looking for plant foods to replace animal products. Not surprisingly, proponents of low-carb and omnivorous diets have responded with a barrage of anti-soy literature.

After many years of tracking the soy wars, I have yet to encounter evidence that would compel me to whole-heartedly embrace or summarily reject soy products. My conclusion is that the right kind and proper amount of soy as part of a well-balanced diet can be beneficial for some individuals, while others might be better off without it. Here are the details:

## Toxins and Antinutrients
Soy beans contain several substances which are the focal point of controversy:

- **Allergens.** Soy protein is one of the top eight allergens. However, it is close to the bottom of that list, while milk, eggs and peanuts are toward the top of the list.[1]
- **Saponins.** Saponins are reputed to lower cholesterol, but can also irritate the lining of the intestines.
- **Protease inhibitors.** Like all seeds, soybeans contain protease inhibitors, which interfere with protein digestion. On the other hand, some authorities claim that these protease inhibitors might actually be beneficial in treating AIDS and reducing infection and inflammation.

- **Phytate** (phytic acid or IP6). This substance pulls minerals, such as calcium, zinc, and iodine, out of the body. On the other hand, the same phytate seems to be useful for pulling toxic metals out of the body, as well as fighting heart disease and certain cancers. Phytate is found in all seeds but is especially high in soybeans.
- **Isoflavones** are phytoestrogens (plant estrogens). The most popular form is called *genistein*. Some studies suggest that isoflavones inhibit breast cancers and prevent osteoporosis.[2,3] However, other studies suggest that isoflavones can act as endocrine disruptors and can contribute to infertility and brain degeneration.[4,5]

## Fermented Soy

Much of the reliable evidence linking soy to reduced rates of cancer and heart disease came from Japan, where soy has been traditionally consumed in the form of fermented soy products such as *miso, shoyu* (traditional soy sauce), *tempeh* and *natto*.

Fermentation makes soy more digestible. Fermentation, along with soaking and cooking, reduces the level of the gas-producing carbohydrates. Fermentation also reduces the antinutrients described above. It also creates beneficial substances, including vitamins, antioxidants, and enzymes. For example, one of the enzymes found in natto is called nattokinase, which has been found to break down blood clots and lower blood pressure.

## Tofu and Other Soy Products

Although traditional fermented tofu is a clean and nutritious food, we should bear in mind that it is not a *whole* food. Like cheese, it is a concentrated food extract. Digesting tofu is not unlike digesting pasteurized cheese or cooked meat, requiring a large output of digestive enzymes. In addition, most of the cheap commercially available tofu is not fermented and is made from soy beans that are probably genetically modified and laden with herbicides and pesticides.

Other unfermented soy products include soy flour, soy lecithin and textured vegetable protein (TVP), all of which are a far cry from the traditional fermented soy products described above. In fact, some of the health problems encountered by modern vegetarians and vegans might be attributed to the liberal use of highly processed soy products, as well as the overuse of soy in general. In contrast, vegetarian or near-vegetarian societies that show good health and longevity typically consume an abundance of produce, along with whole grains, a variety of whole legumes, and starchy vegetables.

Furthermore, much of the commercially produced soybeans in the U.S. are genetically modified and sprayed heavily with pesticides and herbicides. In fact, GMO soy beans have been modified to tolerate larger doses of herbicide, which means that when you eat those beans, you get the double whammy of genetic modification and higher levels of herbicide residue.

**Conclusion**

I am inclined to think that your body is telling you right now, even as you read this passage, if soy is a good food for you. If your inner guide gives soy a nod, I would also suggest that you favor traditional fermented soy made from organically or naturally grown whole soybeans — and let it be part of an overall diet that includes other legumes.

If tofu is appealing to you, eat it in moderation, as you would other concentrated non-whole foods. Remember, a good food can become a bad food if you overconsume it. Tofu is especially easy to overconsume because it is cheap, versatile, and easy to prepare.

Tofu and other processed soy products, such as veggie hot dogs, burgers, and various other products made from textured vegetable protein, have become the fast-foods of the vegetarian world. In general, health-promoting food is not fast food. It is not heavily processed food. Health food is typically slow food. It is whole food.

Bottom line: If you feel drawn to eat soy, avoid overusing it, and take the time to prepare nutritious "slow food," rather than habitually grabbing the tofu or other soy-based fast foods. Make a delicious black bean burger, or a TLT (tempeh, lettuce, and tomato) sandwich. Enjoy a simple and delicately spiced bowl of rice and lentils, with a side dish of sautéed or steamed vegetables. When you eat tofu, do so as in the traditional Asian diets — combined with a generous helping of vegetables, and include sea vegetation, such as nori or wakame.

# Appendix C
# Is Salt Bad for You?

Over the years, I have seen patients with various health issues that showed improvement by reducing their salt intake. However, I have never advised anyone to eliminate added salt, except as a temporary measure.

I personally do not add salt to my food on most days, and I tend to avoid foods that already have added salt. On the days that I do add salt to my food, I have learned to be careful, because if I go beyond a pinch, I might experience disturbed sleep. On the other hand, I have also seen evidence suggesting that some salt is not merely okay, but beneficial and perhaps even necessary for some individuals.[1]

In other words, some individuals seem to benefit from ingesting more salt than we normally encounter in naturally-occurring foods. For example, while I was putting the finishing touches on this book, a friend and colleague shared with me the following information regarding salt restriction:

> Published research has reported that for people with elevated blood pressure, salt restricted diets lowered blood pressure by only one to seven points. However, increasing calcium and potassium does make a significant difference. In addition, as potassium is increased, so does sodium excretion.[2,3] Another study showed that individuals who were put on low salt diets experienced insulin resistance. However, other individuals didn't seem to have that effect.[4,5] No one seems to be able to figure out why some individuals become insulin resistant, and others don't.
>
> I personally learned about the dangers of a relatively low sodium diet about 10 years ago when I was told that my kidneys were failing rapidly, and if I did not cut way back on my protein intake, I would be on dialysis in three years with a very short life expectancy. A medical doctor told me to use only pink sea salt, and to increase my salt intake to 1/4 tsp per glass of water, with a minimum of 6 to 7 glasses per day. He said that he had given this advice to other kidney patients and all but two recovered. I took his advice and my kidneys improved significantly within a month and were all better within three months. I haven't needed to see a nephrologist since.[6]

The information shared above reminds me that the common practice of adding salt to food has become yet another area of controversy in the nutritional world. To bring some clarity to this subject, let's apply some of the principles described in this book:

## Favor Whole Foods

To fully appreciate why we should be conservative with salt, we need only remember that it is not a whole food. It is essentially a highly concentrated, isolated nutrient.

The body is designed to receive nutrients in whole food form, wherein each nutrient is synergistically combined with other nutrients. The use of non-whole foods and isolated nutrients, such as salt, is a relatively recent addition to human diets. Prior to that, sodium, like other minerals, was obtained from food.

As the use of non-whole foods increases, synergy is lost. Furthermore, when we consume any nutrient in amounts that exceed the levels encountered in whole foods, it may no longer simply act as a nutrient that helps maintain normal physiology, but rather can alter physiology — often for the worse. For example, though some studies suggest that low levels of sodium can trigger insulin resistance, other studies indicate that high levels of sodium can do the same. In addition, sodium can act as a stimulant, as well as inhibiting the dilation of arteries.[7,8] Therefore, one of the principles for healthy eating is to fulfill as much of our nutritional requirements as we can with whole foods, while being conservative with extracted foods and isolated nutrients, such as tofu, cheese, coconut oil, butter, and salt.

## Good Nutrition is about Relationship

The effect of a given amount of sodium depends on the other nutrients which happen to be present. For example, the effect that a given amount of dietary sodium has on blood pressure depends on how much calcium and potassium are also present. Higher levels of potassium cause the body to excrete sodium, and vice versa. Therefore, trying to adjust our potassium and sodium intake by using added salt and supplemental potassium is like walking a tight-rope. It should be done with great care, especially for someone with cardiovascular or kidney issues.

For those who do not have heart or kidney issues, a simpler approach is to include foods high in potassium. The highest food sources are listed in Appendix D.

One of the benefits of basing your diet on whole foods with an ample amount of produce, is that the body is more likely to give you accurate signals regarding anything else that you might need to complete your nutritional picture — such as a pinch of salt.

To fully appreciate the balancing power of fruits and vegetables, we need only remember that they do more than just provide potassium. They have other minerals, as well as vitamins and phytonutrients, all synergistically blended by Mother Nature. These other micronutrients contribute to the natural favor and satiating power of food, so we are not so dependent on added salt as our default flavor enhancer. Instead, salt can be used more thoughtfully to add sodium that is genuinely needed. Under such circumstances, the average person can probably just rely on his or her taste buds to regulate salt intake.

## Good Nutrition is not One-size-fits-all

If humanity consisted of a small band of healthy and genetically homogenous individuals living in the Garden of Eden, we would be able to get all the sodium we needed from a wide variety of high-quality whole foods grown on mineral-rich soil. However, things have obviously changed. Eons have passed since the great diaspora when our common ancestors left their primordial forest home and diversified to adapt to various climates, lifestyles, and foods. We must bear this in mind when we make generalities about human nutrition.

Are you one of the individuals who can benefit from adding salt to food? Or, are you just "addicted" to salt? In my opinion, *you* are ultimately the best judge of that. I am also inclined to think that if you are like most individuals, you need only quiet your mind, listen to your body, and trust your judgment and taste buds to determine how much added salt is appropriate for you.

Naturally, if you have high blood pressure or kidney issues, I would also encourage you to consult with a qualified health professional about your sodium needs. As for the official guidelines given by government health authorities, they do provide a useful reference point, but should be taken "with a grain of salt."

# Appendix D
# Common Foods Rich in Potassium

Daily Recommended Intake: 4700 milligrams.

| Food | Mg of Potassium |
| --- | --- |
| 1 med baked potato w skin | 925 |
| 1 med baked sweet potato w skin | 450 |
| 1 medium raw tomato | 290 |
| ½ cup of mushrooms | 280 |
| ½ cup of fresh Brussels sprouts | 250 |
| ½ cup of squash | 250 |
| ¼ of a medium avocado | 245 |
| ½ cup of broccoli | 230 |
| ½ cup of corn | 195 |
| ½ cup of fresh or cooked carrots | 180 |
| ½ cup of asparagus | 155 |
| ½ cup of prune juice | 370 |
| ¼ cup of raisins | 270 |
| 1 medium mango | 325 |
| 1 kiwi fruit | 240 |
| 1 small orange | 240 |
| ½ cup of cubed cantaloupe | 215 |
| 1 medium pear | 200 |

# Appendix E
# Is Coconut Oil Good for *You?*

To place coconut oil into perspective, we must first remember that it is an *oil*. Ingesting coconut oil that you buy from the store is not the same as opening a fresh coconut, eating the meat, and then washing it down with the fresh coconut water. In short, coconut oil is not a whole food. It a highly concentrated food extract.

Since coconut oil has been removed from its whole-food matrix, the calories have become very concentrated, while the other nutritional elements which help the body to process those calories have been removed. With such a product, overconsumption of calories is easy because our natural eating instincts cannot regulate it as well as whole coconut. For example, if we crack open and eat a fresh coconut and manage to eat the whole thing, we will probably not want to eat another one, because the brain will have had enough time to get the signal that the stomach has just received a large dose of calories. In fact, we might feel inclined to stop eating the coconut before finishing it.

In other words, we can pretty much rely on our instinctual food radar to tell us when to stop eating fresh coconut. However, coconut *oil* is another story. Ingesting 1-3 tablespoons of coconut oil in one dose first thing in the morning is easy. Later that same day, we might also use coconut oil to fry or sauté food, well as adding it to smoothies and other prepared foods. Over the course of the day, and with very little effort, we may consume 6 hundred or more calories of coconut oil alone. Therefore, the rule of thumb for using coconut oil (or any extracted oil) is to be mindful of quantity.

## Saturated Fat

Critics of coconut oil claim that it is not a healthy food because it is high in saturated fat. However, the saturated fat in coconut oil is different from the saturated fat found in most animal products. The latter contain mostly long-chain fatty acids which tend to form solid fats. In contrast, coconut oil has more of the medium-chain fatty acids which are solid at room temperature, *but melt at body temperature,* making them easier for to disperse and mingle with the body's watery environment. Furthermore, medium-chain fatty acids burn more easily and efficiently that long-chain fatty acids, making them a source of quick energy, similar to glucose.

Concern about dietary saturated fats centers around its cholesterol elevating effect, especially LDL, as described in chapter 12. In addition, high levels of saturated fats have been linked to insulin resistance.[1,2] Other studies suggest that high levels of saturated fat stiffen arteries.[3] However, there studies were done with saturated fats from animal origin, *not coconut oil.*

How does coconut oil affect cholesterol levels? So far, the studies have been  inconsistent. However, if coconut oil does elevate cholesterol, the studies done thus far suggest that it does not do so as much as the saturated fats from animal origin and might actually improve the overall lipid profiles by elevating HDL.

What are the long-term effects of ingesting coconut oil? Here again, we cannot say if the long-term effects are beneficial, harmful, or neutral, because such studies have yet to be done at a level that would provide an answer. We do have some studies suggesting that long-term use, even in large amounts, might be harmless. However, such studies were done on populations living in tropics. For these folks, fresh coconut (not necessarily coconut oil) was part of their traditional diet for many generations — a diet that also included an abundance of fresh fruits and vegetables.

Though we cannot make any claims for or against ingesting *substantial amounts* of coconut oil as part of our *everyday diet*, we do have evidence that it can have multiple benefits when used conservatively for various therapeutic purposes.[4,5] Here are some of the reported benefits of coconut oil:

- Anti-inflammatory
- Analgesic
- Antifungal
- Used topically, helps to moisturize, and heal skin, and can possibly promote hair growth.
- Has been used to help individuals with Alzheimer's and Parkinson's disease.

# Appendix F
## Enemas & Colonic Irrigations

Enemas and colonic irrigations are two methods of rapidly cleaning out the rectum and colon. They have been used by physicians and other healers throughout the world for literally thousands of years. Though both have been marginalized by modern medicine, they are now receiving more attention.

### The High Enema

The high enema is done with 1-2 quarts of warm clean water, gradually introduced into the rectum. There is disagreement regarding the benefits and safety of doing enemas. The benefit is that it can quickly eliminate a log-jam of putrefying debris. This, in turn, is believed to assist the body in healing and tonifying the large intestine and restoring normal function.

A draw-back is that excessive use can result in loss of minerals and beneficial bacteria. Another draw-back is that some of the water which is introduced into the large intestine can mingle with the residue to form a toxic "tea" that can seep into the blood — especially if the body is already dehydrated.

Are enemas necessary? More specifically, do the benefits outweigh the drawbacks? Opinions vary among health professionals. My conclusion is that the potential value of enemas varies from one individual to the next.

The proper use of enemas starts with the understanding of how we normally keep the large intestine clean and healthy. Quite simply, we eliminate intestinal waste by gently pushing it out from above — by including adequate fiber in the diet, exercising, and taking care to be well-hydrated. However, if the large intestine becomes so congested and devitalized that it is obviously having a hard time pushing things out from above, occasional washing from below might be beneficial as part of an overall program for gently cleansing and healing the body.

Are enemas for you? I believe you are ultimately the best judge of that. If you are not sure, consult with a trusted health professional who is familiar with your physical condition and can guide you in doing the procedure safely and effectively.

**Colonic Irrigations** (Colon hydrotherapy)

Colon hydrotherapy can clean the large intestine more thoroughly than several flushes with an enema bag. However, virtually all available data on the benefits of colon hydrotherapy is anecdotal – testimonials from users and reports from health professionals after years of clinical practice. It is reported to have a number of benefits: mood elevation, improved concentration, and more energy; relieving constipation and allergies; improvement of skin conditions, asthma, and bronchitis; weight loss; headaches.

The potential draw-backs side effects are loss of minerals, nausea, and risk of perforation or infection. What is the likelihood of encountering these adverse reactions? Unfortunately, we still do not have enough hard data on this subject. What we can say is that the reported benefits been significant enough – and the reported adverse reactions small and infrequent enough – to compel local governments to legally recognize colon hydrotherapy.

The main concern with colon hydrotherapy is the self-administered home units, rather than treatments performed by trained therapists.[2] One study reported that 5,600 colon irrigations were done each month in the UK, with no serious side effects.[3] The same claim cannot be made for prescription and non-prescription drugs.[4] In other words, the risk of serious complications, such as perforation of the large intestine, appears to be quite small, especially if the procedure is done by a trained therapist. In contrast, the incidence of perforation during a medical colonoscopy is significant enough to merit close study.[5]

Colon hydrotherapy is now offered by various health care providers, including medical doctors. Training and certification in this procedure is readily available. On the legal side, most states in the United States and many other countries either quietly allow or actively regulate colon hydrotherapy.

In summary, though more scientific study is needed, colon hydrotherapy appears to be a useful resource for individuals with various health issues. However, the procedure poses enough risk that it is best administered by skilled therapists. If you choose to do colon hydrotherapy at home, educate yourself on its proper use. As with enemas, the rule of thumb is to use colon hydrotherapy conservatively and judiciously as part of an overall program that includes good nutrition, exercise, and adequate hydration.

# Appendix G
# Coffee: Good to the Last Drop?

Coffee has benefits but can also be problematic. The main issue with coffee is the stimulating effect of caffeine. The repeated "lift" of caffeine makes it easy to forget that it is an irritant! The body responds to the presence of irritants by activating the adrenal glands, which upregulate our metabolism, so the body can dispose of the irritant as quickly as possible. However, to put the toxicity of caffeine into perspective, we should remember that its lethal dose is roughly 10 grams, which translates into about 75 cups of coffee. The real question is, what are the long-term effects of regular coffee consumption? The answer is not as simple as good or bad.

Yes, caffeine tends to be addictive, which is reason enough to be cautious with it. We should also remember that coffee is often just one of several sources of caffeine available us. Other sources include artificial caffeine products. Caffeine is the most widely used drug in the world.[1] At this juncture, we should also add that such concentrated forms of factory-made caffeine are a far cry from the relatively modest doses found in natural sources, such as coffee and green tea.

On the positive side, caffeine from natural sources is often accompanied by other nutrients that help the body metabolize the caffeine and might actually combine with it to produce some of the reported benefits of these products. Some studies show an inverse relation between coffee consumption and the incidence of various degenerative diseases, as described in the table on the next page.

There are even health practitioners who claim that coffee enemas have health benefits. This would add new meaning to the term, "Good to the last drop," but all humor aside, the internet abounds with testimonials regarding the health benefits of coffee enemas, including for cancer treatment.[2] The claims include the assertion that coffee enemas can upregulate the production of glutathione transferase, thus promoting deep detoxification and liver cleaning. These claims have yet to be substantiated by formal studies, but we should not be quick to dismiss them just because we have no hard science to support them. We do have anecdotal clinical data from that support the therapeutic use of coffee enemas. And formal studies *do* exist which suggest that drinking coffee can have multiple health benefits, including possible anticancer properties, as described in the table that follows. This table summarizes the documented pros and cons of coffee. After you read it, let your own common sense and instincts tell you if coffee is for you. How much should you drink? Here again, I believe you are the best judge of that.

| The downside of Coffee | The upside of Coffee |
|---|---|
| Caffeine causes release of stress hormones, which can have multiple negative effects, as described in chapter 9. | Though the cortisol raising effects of caffeine are cause for concern, studies suggest that drinking coffee can have benefits |
| Caffeine causes tight muscles, anxiety, and insomnia. What's more, studies show that when coffee drinkers abstain for a while, muscle tension and anxiety increase even more.[3] | Though high levels of caffeine can cause muscle tightness and anxiety, studies show that moderate coffee use during and after exercise improve performance and reduce post work out muscle soreness.[4] |
| Caffeine can promote calcium loss which could contribute to osteoporosis.[5] | Though caffeine can cause calcium excretion, evidence linking coffee with osteoporosis is inconsistent.[5] |
| Caffeine delays stomach emptying.[6] | Coffee can relieve constipation.[6] |
| High levels of caffeine raise cortisol levels, which can kill brain cells.[7] | Though high cortisol kills brain cells, studies show moderate coffee intake improves cognitive function in Parkinson's and Alzheimer's disease. [8] |
| High levels of cafestol and kahweol, both found in coffee, raise serum cholesterol. [9] | Cafesol and kahweol are anti-inflammatory, anti-angiogenic, and promote detoxification; they may protect against cancer and benefit the liver.[9] |
| High cortisol levels can reduce insulin sensitivity and thus contribute to type 2 diabetes, as described in chapter 15. | Though high cortisol reduces insulin sensitivity, regular coffee consumption has been associated with lower rates of type 2 diabetes mellitus.[10] |

# Appendix H
# How Much Vitamin C Do *You* Need?

The first historical evidence for the great importance of vitamin C was the death of sailors centuries ago from a disease called scurvy. Individuals with this condition suffer from extremely brittle bones and fragile blood vessels, making them very vulnerable to fractures and hemorrhage. For example, an individual with an advanced case of scurvy might experience a broken jaw from just chewing food. The same individuals might also bruise very easily and have severe nose bleeds and bleeding gums.

A British physician eventually discovered that giving sailors oranges, lemons, or limes prevented scurvy — that is why British sailors were later called "Limeys." Much later, in the 1930s, research showed that scurvy is the result of a severe vitamin C deficiency.

The official recommended daily intake (RDI) for vitamin C is currently set at 75 mg for adult females and 90 mg for adult males. However, according to human and animal studies, these numbers are probably much too low.

The vast majority of animals make their own vitamin C. How much do they make? Adjusted to human weight, they make the equivalent of thousands of milligrams per day.[1] Primates (monkeys, apes, and humans) are the only major group of animals that do not make their own vitamin C. How much vitamin C do monkeys and apes get in the wild? Adjusted to human weight, they get thousands of milligrams per day.[2]

We can easily why primates in the wild would not have to make vitamin C – the main sources of vitamin C are fresh fruits and vegetables. Primates in the wild eat mostly fruits and vegetables. With an abundance of fresh fruits and vegetables, primates in the wild easily maintain blood levels of vitamin C which are about ten times that of most humans.

## Animals in the wild do not Get Heart Attacks

Research suggests that vitamin C might be one factor which accounts for the virtual absence of cardiovascular disease in wild animals, while the same disease is the main cause of death in modern humans.[3] For example, wild gorillas do not suffer from cardiovascular disease. Neither are they prone to obesity and blood sugar issues. However, gorillas in captivity have been known to develop all these conditions, as well as dying prematurely for no apparent reason. Likewise, such gorillas showed an improvement in health when given levels of vitamin C they would normally receive in the wild. This is consistent with human studies that link low levels of vitamin C with a number of health issues, such as high cholesterol, cardiovascular disease, bleeding gums, bruising, strokes, excess fat storage, asthma, greater susceptibility to respiratory infections, low energy, fatigue, rapid aging of tissues and cancer.

When we combine the above data with the many known functions of vitamin C, we can see why the official RDI might be way too low, especially for individuals who wish to prevent or recover from various illnesses.

## Functions of vitamins C
- It is a major anti-oxidant.
- It is needed to make collagen, the glue that holds the body together. Therefore, it is essential for maintaining the integrity of virtually all tissues, and for recovery from injury.
- Since collagen is a major component of blood vessels, vitamin C is essential for maintaining the integrity of blood vessels.
- Helps to eliminate viruses, bacteria, and cancer cells.
- Modulates the immune system to reduce allergic reactions.

## Signs of Vitamin C Deficiencies
- Allergies
- Frequent colds and flu
- Weak tendons and ligaments, and brittle bones
- Increased fractures and injury to muscles and joints
- Poor wound healing and regeneration
- Hemorrhaging, such as bleeding gums, nose bleeds and bruising
- Cardiovascular disease, strokes, cancer, and arthritis

## For Optimum Health
For optimum health, some health authorities suggest 1000 mg of vitamin C per day. In fact, the studies cited above suggest that even higher levels may be appropriate. Higher levels can be achieved by including fresh produce that is especially rich in vitamin C, as shown in the following page.

| Food | Vit C levels per lb of food |
|---|---|
| Yellow bell peppers | 832 mg |
| Red bell peppers | 579 |
| Kale | 544 |
| Kiwi | 420 |
| Brussels sprouts | 386 |
| Papaya | 276 |
| Strawberries | 267 |
| Oranges | 241 |
| Lemons | 240 |
| Pineapples | 217 |
| Grapefruit | 172 |
| Mangos | 165 |
| Spinach | 128 |
| Raspberries | 119 |
| Blackberries | 95 |
| Tomatoes | 62 |
| Blueberries | 44 |

Studies suggest that vitamin C tends to be more effective when obtained from food sources.[4] This may be due to the fact that the vitamin C in food is synergistically combined with other nutrients. Pure vitamin C is ascorbic acid. In foods, ascorbic acid is found in combination with other substances, such as flavonoids, rutin and hesperidin. Together, they make up the so-called C complex.

We should also bear in mind that the need for vitamin C increases with any kind of stress, especially infections and increased toxic burden. Under such circumstances, the right kind of supplementation can be beneficial. In fact, very large doses of vitamin C, usually pure ascorbic acid, have been used therapeutically, sometimes intravenously, to help patients recover from serious illness.

# Appendix I
# The Glycemic Index

The glycemic index is a measure of how readily a given food sends glucose into the blood. There are two ways of measuring the glycemic index. One system uses white flour as the basis of reference by which to evaluate other foods. Another system uses pure glucose as the reference. In the latter system, the index ranges from 0 to 100. Pure glucose has the maximum value of 100. Using this system, the glycemic index of a given food is evaluated as follows:

| Classification | Range | Examples |
| --- | --- | --- |
| Low GI | 55 or less | Most fruits and vegetables, grainy breads, brown rice, legumes, milk, fish, eggs, meat, some cheeses, and nuts |
| Medium GI | 56 – 69 | Whole wheat products, basmati rice, sweet potatoes |
| High GI | 70 and above | Corn flakes, baked potato, croissants, white bread, most cold breakfast cereals |

In the above list, notice that the higher glycemic foods are cooked starchy foods and products made with refined sugars. These are the same foods that are often combined with concentrated fatty foods, resulting in blood sugar chaos.

Some nutritional authorities advise caution about placing too much weight on the glycemic index to evaluate a given food, because other factors, such as the presence of soluble fiber, vitamins, minerals, and phytonutrients, may be more important in determining how that food will influence blood sugar. In general, however, individuals with blood sugar issues are well-advised to favor lower glycemic foods.

# Endnotes and References

## Chapter 1

1. Goralczyk R. Beta-carotene and lung cancer in smokers: review of hypotheses and status of research. Nutr Cancer. 2009;61(6):767-74.
2. Podmore ID, et al. Vitamin C exhibits pro-oxidant properties. Nature. 1998 Apr 9;392(6676):559.
3. Pollan, M. The Omnivores Dilemma. 147-148. Penguin Press, 2006.
4. Pollan, M. The Omnivores Dilemma. 150-151. Penguin Press, 2006.
5. In recent years, the emerging field of Epigenetics has revealed that that gene expression can be profoundly influenced by environmental factors – including food. For example, the foods eaten by the pregnant mother can influence genetic expression in the baby.

## Chapter 2

1. Pollan, M. Food Rules. The Penguin Press, 2011.
2. Fleet. T. Rays of the Dawn. Pgs 13-15. Thurmond Fleet, 1948

## Chapter 3

1. Cataloging foods as pro and anti-inflammatory is useful as long as we do not interpret it to mean that one is good and the other bad. The so-called proinflammatory foods have the *potential* to stimulate inflammation when overconsumed and not balanced with anti-inflammatory foods. The latter have features that support the body in having an inflammatory response that remains in the ideal "Goldie Locks" zone — not too much not too little.
2. Kiecolt-Glaser, JK. Stress, Food, and Inflammation: psychoneuroimmunology and Nutrition at the Cutting Edge. Psychosom Med. 2010 May; 72(4): 365–369.
3. Singh B, et al. Bioactive compounds in banana and their associated health benefits - A review. Food Chem. 2016 Sep 1;206:1-11.
4. Aviram M, et al. Pomegranate juice consumption for 3 years by patients with carotid artery stenosis reduces common carotid intima-media thickness, blood pressure and LDL oxidation. Clin Nutr. 2004 Jun;23(3):423-33.
5. Li. T, et al. Usefulness of pumpkin seeds combined with areca nut extract in community-based treatment of human taeniasis in NW Sichuan Province, China. Acta Trop. 2012 Nov;124(2):152-7.
6. Pathak N, et al. Value addition in sesame: A perspective on bioactive components for enhancing utility and profitability. Pharmacogn Rev. 2014 Jul-Dec; 8(16): 147–155.
7. Mericil F, et al. Fatty acid composition and anticancer activity in colon carcinoma cell lines of Prunus dulcis seed oil. Pharm Biol. 2017 Dec;55(1):1239-1248.

# Chapter 4

1. Parkman HP. et al. Cholecystectomy and Clinical Presentations of Gastroparesis. Digestive Diseases and Sciences. April 2013, Volume 58, Issue 4, pp 1062–1073
2. Dongyeop L. et al. Effects of nutritional components on aging. Aging Cell. 2015 Feb; 14(1): 8–16.
3. Friedman AN. High-protein diets: potential effects on the kidney in renal health and disease. Am J Kidney Dis. 2004 Dec;44(6):950-62.
4. Solberg, E. et al. Stress reactivity to and recovery from a standardized exercise bout: a study of 31 runners practicing relaxation techniques. Br J Sports Med 2000;34:268-272.
5. Ippokratis P, et al. Do Nonsteroidal Anti-Inflammatory Drugs Affect Bone Healing? A Critical Analysis. ScientificWorldJournal. 2012; 2012: 606404.
6. Coutinho, A. E. and Chapman, K.E. The anti-inflammatory and immunosuppressive effects of glucocorticoids, recent developments, and mechanistic insights. Mol Cell Endocrinol. 2011 Mar 15; 335(1): 2–13.
7. Esmaeilzadeh F. Does Intermittent Fasting Improve Microvascular Endothelial Function in Healthy Middle-aged Subjects? Published on line Sept 14, 2016: Biology and Medicine (website).
8. Honjoh, S. et al. Signaling through RHEB-1 mediated intermittent fasting-induced longevity in C. elegans. Nature 457, 726-730 (5 February 2009).
9. McCoy, F. The Fast Way to Heal. McCoy Publ 1926
10. Brandt, J. The Grape Cure. Beneficial Books 1967
11. Tripp, D. How Intermittent Fasting Might Help You Live a Longer and Healthier Life. Scientific American. Jan 2013.
12. One such facility is the True North Health Center, in Santa Rosa, California.

# Chapter 5

1. Whorton, J. Medical Myth. Civilization and the colon Constipation
2. as "the disease of diseases" West J Med. 2000 Dec; 173(6): 424–427.
3. Ernst E. Colonic irrigation and the theory of autointoxication: a triumph of ignorance over science. J Clin Gastroenterol. 1997 Jun;24(4):196-8.
4. Hughes R., et al. Protein degradation in the large intestine: Relevance to colorectal cancer. Curr. Issues in Intestinal Microbiol. 2000; 1:51–58.
5. Toden S, et al. Resistant starch attenuates colon DNA damage induced by high dietary protein in rats. Nutr. Cancer. 2005;51:45–51.
6. Löser C, et el. Polyamines in colorectal cancer. Evaluation of polyamine concentrations in colon tissue, serum, and urine of 50 patients with colorectal cancer. Cancer. 1990 Feb 15;65(4):958-66.

7. Moreira A.P.B., et al. Influence of high-fat diet on gut microbiota, intestinal permeability and metabolic endotoxaemia. Br. J. Nutr. 2012;108:801–809.
8. Ou J., de Lany J.P., Zhang M., Sharma S., O'Keefe S.J.D. Association between low colonic short-chain fatty acids and high bile acids in high colon cancer risk populations. Nutr. Cancer. 2012;64:34–40.
9. Ridlon J.M., Kang D.-J., Hylemon P.B. Bile salt biotransformations by human intestinal bacteria. J. Lipid Res. 2006;47:241–259.
10. Weil, A. Natural Health, Natural Medicine. The Complete Guide to Wellness and Self Care for Optimum Health. Houghton Mifflin Company, 2004.
11. Sear, M Chelation: Harnessing and Enhancing Heavy Metal detoxification. Scientific WorldJournal. 2013; 2013: 219840.
12. Walker, M. Medical Journalist Report of Innovative Biologics. Value of Colon Hydrotherapy verified by medical professionals prescribing it. Townsend Letter for Doctors & Patients: August / September 2000 (#205/206).
13. Michalsen, A. et al. Mediterranean diet or extended fasting's influence on changing the intestinal microflora, immunoglobulin A secretion and clinical outcome in patients with rheumatoid arthritis and fibromyalgia: an observational study. BMC Complement Altern Med. 2005; 5: 22.

# Chapter 6

1. Conlon, M.A., Anthony R. Bird, A.,R. The Impact of Diet and Lifestyle on Gut Microbiota and Human, Nutrients. 2015 Jan; 7(1): 17–44.
2. Sear. Cynthia L. Garret, W. Microbes, Microbiota and Colon Cancer. Cell Host Microbe. 2014 Mar 12; 15(3): 317–328.
3. Angélica T. et al. The Role of Probiotics and Prebiotics in Inducing Gut Immunity. Frontier of Immunology. 2013; 4: 445.
4. Justyna Bien, Vindhya Palagani, and Przemyslaw Bozko. The intestinal microbiota dysbiosis and *Clostridium difficile* infection: is there a relationship with inflammatory bowel disease? Therap Adv Gastroenterol. 2013 Jan; 6(1): 53–68.
5. Albert MJ, Mathan VI, Baker SJ. Vitamin $B_{12}$ synthesis by human small intestinal bacteria. Nature. 1980; 283 (Feb 21):781-2.
6. Liu Z, et al. Tight junctions, leaky intestines, and pediatric diseases. Acta Paediatrica. 2005 Apr;94(4):386-93.
7. Bischoff SC., et al. Intestinal permeability – a new target for disease prevention and therapy. BMC Gastroenterol. 2014; 14: 189.
8. Arriesta MC, et al. Alterations in intestinal permeability. Gut. 2006 Oct; 55(10): 1512–1520.
9. Kelly J, et al. Breaking down the barriers: the gut microbiome, intestinal permeability, and stress-related psychiatric disorders. Front Cell Neurosci. 2015; 9: 392.

10. Shah E, et al. Psychological disorders in gastrointestinal disease: epiphenomenon, cause, or consequence? Ann Gastroenterol. 2014; 27(3): 224–230.
11. Fasano A1. Leaky gut and autoimmune diseases. Clin Rev Allergy Immunol. 2012 Feb;42(1):71-8.
12. Gaby, A. A Review of the Fundamentals of Diet. Glob Adv Health Med. 2013 January; 2(1): 58–63.
13. Kaslow. J. Food Combining. Website: drk.com. Compilation of the clinical results and published works of Howard Hay, M.D., Daniel C. Monro, M.D., L.M. Rogers, M.D. and George Goodheart, D.C.
14. From website: gapsdiet.com.
15. Bone broth is exactly what it sounds like — a broth made from bone, as well as cartilage and marrow.
16. Monro JA, et al. The risk of lead contamination in bone broth diets. Med Hypotheses. 2013 Apr;80(4):389-90.
17. Rapin, J., et al. Possible Links between Intestinal Permeability and Food Processing: A Potential Therapeutic Niche for Glutamine. Clinics (Sao Paulo). 2010 Jun; 65(6): 635–643.
18. Pizzaro L. Highlights from the Institute for Functional Medicine's 2014 Conference: Functional Perspectives on Food and Nutrition: Ultimate Upstream Medicine. Integr Med2014 Oct; 13(5): 38–50.
19. Nagpal R., et al. Effect of Aloe vera juice on growth and activities of Lactobacilli in-vitro. Acta Biomed. 2012 Dec;83(3):183-8.

## Chapter 7

1. Pichichero, M.E. Strep Throat-Recurrent. University of Rochester Medical Center. (from website).
2. Benjamin J. et al. The Gut-Lung Axis in Respiratory Disease. Annals of the American Thoracic Society, Vol. 12, # 2, nov 1.
3. Mahmoud Y.I. Grape seed extract attenuates lung parenchyma pathology in ovalbumin-induced mouse asthma model: an ultrastructural study. Micron. 2012.04.014.
4. Xie XH, et al. Resveratrol Inhibits respiratory syncytial virus-induced IL-6 production, decreases viral replication, and downregulates TRIF expression in airway epithelial cells. Inflammation. 2012 Aug;35(4):1392-401.

## Chapter 8

1. In the past, the role of the skin in respiration was thought to be so critically important that a person could suffocate if the skin was prevented from "breathing" sufficiently. This was found to be not true. However, the skin does directly absorb atmospheric oxygen.
2. Boutin AT., et al. Epidermal sensing of oxygen is essential for systemic hypoxic response. Cell. 2008 Apr 18;133(2):223-34.

3. Rele AS Mohile RB. Effect of mineral oil, sunflower oil, and coconut oil on prevention of hair damage. J Cosmet Sci. 2003 Mar-Apr;54(2):175-92.
4. Khayel G, et al. Effects of fish oil supplementation on inflammatory acne. Lipid Health Dis. Dec11, 2012.
5. Black, H.S., and Rhodes, L.E. Potential Benefits of Omega-3 Fatty Acids in Non-Melanoma Skin Cancer. J Clin Med. 2016 Feb; 5(2): 23.

## Chapter 9

1. Eggleston DW. The Interrelationship of Stress and Degenerative Diseases. Prosthet Dent. 1980. Nov;44(5):541-4.
2. Lyon P, Cohen M, Quintner J. An Evolutionary Stress-Response Hypothesis for Chronic Widespread Pain (Fibromyalgia Syndrome). Pain Med. 2011 Jun 21. doi: 10.1111/j.1526-4637.2011.01168.
3. Selye, Hans. The Stress of Life. New York: McGraw-Hill, 1956.
4. Bracha HS, et al. Does "Fight or Flight" Need Updating? *Psy*chosomatics 45 (5): 448–9.
5. In the 1930s, Paul Kouchakoff MD of Switzerland found that food heated at high temperatures or processed caused a rise in white blood cells. The strongest triggers of this reaction were processed and refined foods such as pasteurized and homogenized milk and margarine, chocolate, refined sugar, candy, white flour, and table salt. In other words, he found that cooked and processed food had a tendency to trigger a low-grade physiological response that resembled the body's response to pathogens and toxins. Interestingly, when the meal included about 15% raw food, the stress response did not occur.
6. Meredith, SE. et al. A Comprehensive Review and Research Agenda. J Caffeine Res. 2013 Sep; 3(3): 114–130.
7. Álvarez-Lario B, Alonso-Valdivielso JL. Hyperuricemia and gout; the role of diet. Nutr Hosp. 2014 Apr 1;29(4):760-70.
8. Blaylock, Russell L. Health and Nutrition Secrets that can Save Your Life. 356. Albuquerque, NM. Health Press, 2006.

## Chapter 10

1. Lyon P, Cohen M, Quintner J. An Evolutionary Stress-Response Hypothesis for Chronic Widespread Pain (Fibromyalgia Syndrome). Pain Med. 2011 Jun 21. doi: 10.1111/j.1526-4637.2011.01168.
2. Branco J, Atalaia A, Paiva T. Sleep cycles and alpha-delta sleep in fibromyalgia syndrome. J Rheumatol. 1994 Jun;21(6):1113-7.
3. Roizenblatt S. Et al. Alpha sleep characteristics in fibromyalgia. Arthritis & Rheumatology, 25 January 2001.
4. Levine ME. Et at. Low Protein Intake Is Associated with a Major Reduction in IGF-1, Cancer, and Overall Mortality in the 65 and Younger but Not Older Population. Cell Metabolism. Vol 19, issue 3, p407-17, March 2014.,

5. Blaylock, Russell L. Health and Nutrition Secrets that can Save Your Life. 356. Albuquerque, NM. Health Press, 2006.
6. Russell IJ, et al. Treatment of fibromyalgia syndrome with Super Malic: a randomized, double blind, placebo controlled, crossover pilot study. J Rheumatol. 1995 May;22(5):953-8.

## Chapter 11

1. Shah SK, Gecy GT. Prednisone-induced osteoporosis: an overlooked and undertreated adverse effect. Journal of the American Osteopath Assoc. 2006 Nov; 106(11):653-7.
2. Domazetovic V., et al. Oxidative stress in bone remodeling: role of antioxidants. Clin Cases Miner Bone Metab. 2017 May-Aug; 14(2): 209–216.
3. Billard CB. High osteoporosis risk among East Africans linked to lactase persistence genotype. Bonekey Reports. 2016 5, article # 803.
4. Batey LA, et al. Skeletal health in adult patients with classic galactosemia. Osteoporos Int. 2013 Feb;24(2):501-9.
5. Lanham-New SA. Fruit and vegetables: the unexpected natural answer to the question of osteoporosis prevention? Am J Clin Nutr. 2006 Jun;83(6):1254-5.
6. Shen CL, et al. Fruits and dietary phytochemicals in bone protection. Nutr Res. 2012 Dec;32(12):897-910.
7. Thie NMR. Prasad, N, Major PW. Evaluation of Glucosamine Sulfate Compared to Ibuprofen for the Treatment of Temporomandibular Joint Osteoarthritis: A Randomized Double Blind Controlled 3 Month Clinical Trial. J Rheumatol 2001;28:1347-55)
8. Joanna Bałan, B., et al. Oral administration of *Aloe vera* gel, anti-microbial and anti-inflammatory herbal remedy, stimulates cell-mediated immunity and antibody production in a mouse model. Cent Eur J Immunol. 2014; 39(2): 125–130.

## Chapter 12

1. Esselstyn, Caldwell, B. Prevent and Reverse Heart Disease. 31-32. Every Books. New York. 2007.
2. Abramson J, Wright JM. Are lipid-lowering guidelines evidencebased? Lancet. 2007 Jan 20; 369(9557):168-9
3. Golomb, B. A. M.D., Ph.D, et al. Statin Adverse Effects: A Review of the Literature and Evidence for a Mitochondrial Mechanism. Am J Cardiovasc Drugs. 2008; 8(6): 373–418.
4. Ikeda U. Inflammation and coronary artery disease. Curr Vasc Pharmacol. 2003 Mar;1(1):65-70.
5. Luigi Fontana, Timothy E. Meyer, Samuel Klein, and John O. Holloszy. Long-Term Low-Calorie Low-Protein Vegan Diet and Endurance Exercise are Associated with Low Cardiometabolic Risk.

rejuvenation Research. June 2007, 10(2): 225-234. doi:10.1089/rej.2006.0529.

6. Furhman, J. Fasting and Eating for Health. St. Martin;s Press. 1995. P. 101-3.

7. Donpunha W, et al. Protective Effect of Ascorbic Acid on Cadmium induced Hypertension and vascular Dysfunction in Mice. *Miometals.* 2011 Feb:24(1) 105–15.

8. Steinberg D. Low density lipoprotein oxidation and its pathobiological significance. J Biol Chem.1997;272:20963–20966.

9. Nunez-Cordoba JM, Martinez-Gonzalez MA. Antioxidant Vitamins and Cardiovascular Disease. Curr Top Med Chem. 2011, April 21.

10. Ganguly, P, Sreyoshi Fatima, S. A. Nutr J. 2015; 14: 6. Role of homocysteine in the development of cardiovascular disease.

11. (No authors listed) Randomised trial of cholesterol lowering in 4444 patients with coronary heart disease: the Scandinavian Simvastatin Survival Study (4S). Lancet. 1994 Nov 19;344(8934):1383-9.

12. DuBroff, R, de Lorgeril, M. Cholesterol confusion and statin controversy World J Cardiol. 2015 Jul 26; 7(7): 404–409.

13. Farquhar, WB., et al. Dietary Sodium and Health: More Than Just Blood Pressure. J Am Coll Cardio.2015 March 17; 65(10):1042–1050.

14. Staprans I, et al. Cholesterol in the Diet Accelerates the Development of Aortic Atherosclerosis in Cholesterol-Fed Rabbits. *Arteriosclerosis, Thrombosis, and Vasc Biology.* 1998; 18:977–983.).

15. Tappel A. Heme of consumed red meat can act as a catalyst of oxidative damage and could initiate colon, breast and prostate cancers, heart disease and other diseases. Med Hypotheses. 2007. 68(3):562–4.

16. Vogel, Robert, A. Brachial Artery Ultrasound: A Noninvasive Tool in Assessment of Triglyceride Rich Lipoproteins. *Clinical Cardiology.* June 1999.

17. Holt H, et al. Insulin Index of Foods: insulin demand generated by 100kj portions of common foods. *Am J Cli Nutr.* 1997. 66:1264–1267.

18. Tuso, PJ., et al. Nutritional Update for Physicians: Plant-Based Diets. Perm J. 2013 Spring; 17(2): 61–66.

19. Hu, FB. Plant-based foods and prevention of cardiovascular disease. Am J Clin Nutri. Spt 20033. Vol 78 no. 3544s-551s.

20. Jenkins, JD., et al. Effect of a 6-month vegan low-carbohydrate ('Eco-Atkins') diet on cardiovascular risk factors and body weight in hyperlipidaemic adults: a randomised controlled trial. BMJ Open. 2014 Feb 5;4(2).

21. Kelly JH. Sabaté J. Nuts and coronary heart disease: an epidemiological perspective. Br J Nutr. 2006 Nov;96 Suppl 2:S61-7.

22. Hu FB. Stampfer MJ. Nut consumption and risk of coronary heart disease: a review of epidemiologic evidence. Curr Atheroscler Rep. 1999 Nov;1(3):204-9.

23. Aviram M, et al. Pomegranate juice consumption reduces oxidative stress, atherogenic modifications to LDL, and platelet aggregation. Am J Clin Nutr. 2000 May;71(5):1062-76.
24. Tassell, M. C. et al. Hawthorn (Crataegus spp.) in the treatment of cardiovascular disease. Pharmacogn Rev. 2010 Jan-Jun; 4(7): 32–41.
25. Naderi, G.A. et al. Fibrinolytic effects of Ginkgo biloba extract. Exp Clin Cardiol. 2005 Summer; 10(2): 85–87.
26. Hopkins, A,L, et al. Hibiscus sabdariffa L. in the treatment of hypertension and hyperlipidemia: a comprehensive review of animal and human studies Fitoterapia. 2013 Mar; 85: 84–94.
27. Hsia CH1, et al. Nattokinase decreases plasma levels of fibrinogen, factor VII, and factor VIII in human subjects. Nutr Res. 2009 Mar;29(3):190-6. doi: 10.1016/j.nutres.2009.01.009.
28. Forastiere F, et at. Consumption of Vitamin C in Fresh Fruit and Wheezing Symptoms in Children. SIDRIA Collective Group. Thorax 2000:55(4): 283-8
29. Florea V.G., Cohn, J. N. The Autonomic Nervous System and Heart Failure. Circulation Research. May, 22, 2014.

# Chapter 13

1. Morrow, WJ., et al. Dietary fat and immune function. J Immunol. 1985 Dec;135(6):3857-63.
2. Han Sn, et al. Effect of hydrogenated and saturated, relative to polyunsaturated fat on immune and inflammatory responses of adults with moderate hypercholesterolemia. J Lipid Res. 2002 Mar;43:445-52.
3. Lubick N. immunity: Mercury Alters Immune System Response in Artisanal Gold Miners. Environ Health Perspect. 2010 Jun; 118(6): A243. Bharti V., et al. Fluoride induced oxidative stress, immune system, and apoptosis in animals: a review. International Journal of Bioassays. Nov 2016. 5163.
4. Corsini E. et al. Effects of pesticide exposure on the human immune system. Hum Exp Toxicol. 2008 Sep;27(9):671-80.
5. Fluoride in Drinking Water: A Scientific Review of EPA Standards. National Research council; 2006. National Academic Press. Washington D.C.
6. Akanbi, O, et al. Unexpected outcome (positive or negative) including adverse drug reactions. Antibiotic-associated haemorrhagic colitis: not always Clostridium difficile. BMJ Case Reports 2017.
7. Norgaard M, et at. Use of penicillin and other antibiotics and risk of multiple sclerosis: a population-based case-control study. Am J Epidemiol. 2011 Oct 15;174(8):945-8.
8. McAnulty LS, et al. Effect of blueberry ingestion on natural killer cell counts, oxidative stress, and inflammation prior to and after 2.5 h of

running. Applied Physiology, Nutrition and Metabolism. 2011 Dec;36(6):976-84.

9. Barak V, Halperin T, Kalickman I. The effect of Sambucol, a black elderberry-based, natural product, on the production of human cytokines: I. Inflammatory cytokines. Eur Cytokine Netw. 2001 Apr-Jun;12(2):290-6.

10. Hussain A, et al. Aloe vera inhibits proliferation of human breast and cervical cancer cells and acts synergistically with cisplatin. Asian Pac J Cancer Prev. 2015;16(7):2939-46.

11. Micol V, et al. Antiviral Res. 2005 Jun;66(2-3):129-36. Epub 2005 Apr 18. The olive leaf extract exhibits antiviral activity against viral haemorrhagic septicaemia rhabdovirus (VHSV).Nutrients. 2018 Dec; 10(12): 1950.

12. Russolini J, et al. Oleuropein, the Main Polyphenol of Olea europaea Leaf Extract, Has an Anti-Cancer Effect on Human BRAF Melanoma Cells and Potentiates the Cytotoxicity of Current Chemotherapies. Published online 2018 Dec 8 doi: 10.3390/nu10121950.

13. Swamy MK, et al. Properties of Plant Essential Oils against Human Pathogens and Their Mode of Action. Evid Based Complement Alternat Med. 2016; 2016: 3012462.

14. Huggins MA. Et al. Microbial Exposure Enhances Immunity to Pathogens Recognized by TLR2 but Increases Susceptibility to Cytokine Storm through TLR4 Sensitization. Cell Rep. 2019 Aug 13; 28(7): 1729–1743.e5.

# Chapter 14

1. Some modes of treatment and prevention are emerging which utilize knowledge of the individual's specific genetic predisposition.

2. Abnet, C.C. Carcinogenic Food Contaminants. Cancer Invest. 2007 Apr–May; 25(3): 189–196.

3. Wogan GN, et al. Environmental and chemical carcinogenesis. Semin Cancer Biol. 2004 Dec;14(6):473-86.

4. Nisarg R D., Et al. Pathophysiology of cell phone radiation: oxidative stress and carcinogenesis with focus on male reproductive system. Reprod Biol Endocrinol. 2009; 7: 114.

5. David, A. R.Zimmerman M.R. Cancer: an old disease, a new disease or something in between? Nature Reviews Cancer 10, 728-733 (October 2010).

6. Giovannucci, E. et al. Diabetes and Cancer. Diabetes Care. 2010 Jul; 33(7): 1674–1685.

7. Zhang CX, Ho SC, Chen YM, et al. Greater vegetable, and fruit intake is associated with a lower risk of breast cancer among Chinese women. Int J Cancer 2009;125:181-188.

8. Sun J, et al. Antioxidant and antiproliferative activities of common fruits. J Agric Food Chem. 2002 Dec 4;50(25):7449-54.
9. Rashidkhani B, Lindblad P, Wolk A. Fruits, vegetables, and risk of renal cell carcinoma: a prospective study of Swedish women. Int J Cancer. 2005 Jan 20;113(3):451-5
10. Boivina, D., et al. Antiproliferative and Antioxidant Activity of Common Vegetables. Food Chemistry. Volume 112, Issue 2, 15 January 2009, Pages 374–380.
11. Link, L., Potter, J. Raw versus Cooked Vegetables and Cancer Risk. A review, published by the American Association of Cancer Research. September 2004. (From website).
12. Cohen JH, Kristal AR, Stanford JL. Fruit and vegetable intakes and prostate cancer risk. J Natl Cancer Inst 2000;92:61-68.
13. Higdon J., et al. Cruciferous vegetables, and human cancer risk: epidemiologic evidence and mechanistic basis. Pharmacol Res 2007;55:224-236.
14. Yuan F, Chen DZ, Liu K, et al. Anti-estrogenic activities of indole-3-carbinol in cervical cells: implication for prevention of cervical cancer. Anticancer Res 1999;19:1673-1680.
15. Ramirez MC, Singletary K. Regulation of estrogen receptor alpha expression in human breast cancer cells by sulforaphane. The Journal of nutritional biochemistry 2009;20:195-201.
16. Cornblatt BS, Ye L, Dinkova-Kostova AT, et al. Preclinical and clinical evaluation of sulforaphane for chemoprevention in the breast. Carcinogenesis 2007;28:1485-1490.
17. Wang S., Stoner D. Anthocyanins and their role in cancer prevention. Author mcript; available in PMC 2009 Oct 8.
18. Stoner, GD, et al. Carcinogen-Altered Genes in Rat Esophagus Positively Modulated to Normal Levels of Expression by Both Black Raspberries and Phenylethyl Isothiocyanate. Cancer Res. 2008 Aug 1; 68(15): 6460–6467.
19. McCormack, D., McFadden, D. A Review of Pterostilbene Antioxidant Activity and Disease Modification. Oxid Med Cell Longev. 2013; 2013: 575482.
20. Adams, L S. Phung, S. et al. Blueberry Phytochemicals Inhibit Growth and Metastatic Potential of MDA-MB-231 Breast Cancer Cells Through Modulation of the Phosphatidylinositol 3-Kinase Pathway. Cancer Res. 2010 May 1; 70(9): 3594–3605.
21. Cuevas, A, et al. Modulation of Immune Function by Polyphenols: Possible Contribution of Epigenetic Factors Nutrients. 2013 Jul; 5(7): 2314–2332.
22. Gerhauser C[1]. Cancer chemopreventive potential of apples, apple juice, and apple components. Planta Med. 2008 Oct;74(13):1608-24.

23. Deeba N. et al.  Pomegranate Extracts and Cancer Prevention: Molecular and Cellular Activities.  Anticancer Agents Med Chem. 2013 Oct; 13(8): 1149–1161.
24. Lu QY, et al. Inhibition of prostate cancer cell growth by an avocado extract: role of lipid-soluble bioactive substances. J Nutr Biochem. 2005 Jan;16(1):23-30.
25. Ding H, et al. Selective induction of apoptosis of human oral cancer cell lines by avocado extracts via a ROS-mediated mechanism.
26. Dreher ML. Davenport AJ. Hass Avocado Composition and Potential Health Effects. Crit Rev Food Sci Nutr. 2013 May; 53(7): 738–750.
27. Khan N, Mukhtar H. Cancer and metastasis: prevention and treatment by green tea. Cancer Metastasis Rev. 2010 Sep; 29(3): 435–445.
28. Ji-Yi Hu, et al. Consumption of garlic and risk of colorectal cancer: An updated meta-analysis of prospective studies. Nutr Cancer. 2009;61(3):348-56.
29. Shanmugam MK, et al. The multifaceted role of curcumin in cancer prevention and treatment.  Molecules. 2015 Feb 5;20(2):2728-69.
30. Brown J, et al. Nutrition During and After Cancer Treatment: A Guide* for Informed Choices by Cancer Survivors. CA: A Cancer Journal for Physicians, May 2001.
31. Shaw, NE. Why An Alkaline Approach Can Successfully Treat Cancer. GreenMedInfo LLC, Aug 8, 2013.
32. Mannion C. et al.  Components of an Anticancer Diet: Dietary Recommendations, Restrictions and Supplements of the Bill Henderson Protocol. Nutrients. 2011 Jan; 3(1): 1–26.
33. Finley JW, et al. Cancer-Protective Properties of High-Selenium Broccoli. J. Agric. Food Chem., 2001, 49 (5), pp 2679–2683.
34. Yuesheng Zhang JW, Talalay P. *Broccoli sprouts: An exceptionally rich source of inducers of enzymes that protect against chemical carcinogens. Proc Natl Acad Sci. 1997 Sep 16.94(19): 10367–10372.
35. Eliassen AH, et al. Plasma carotenoids and risk of breast cancer over 20 y of follow-up. Am J Clin Nutr. 2015;101(6):1197-1205.
36. Madreiter-Sokolowski CT, et al. Resveratrol Specifically Kills Cancer Cells by a Devastating Increase in the $Ca^{2+}$ Coupling Between the Greatly Tethered Endoplasmic Reticulum and Mitochondria. Cell Physiol Biochem. 2016;39(4):1404-20.
37. Schaefer, B.A. et al. Nutrition and Cancer: Further Case Studies Involving Salvestrol. JOM Volume 25, Number 1, 2010.
38. Insulin potentiation therapy (IPT) is an experimental form of chemotherapy that uses insulin to enhance absorption of chemotherapy agents by cancer cells. The enhanced absorption allows the drug to be effective at a lower dosage and therefore reduces side effects. Cancer cells have about 20X as many insulin receptors, allowing for rapid glucose absorption. W cancer cells open up to allow glucose to enter, they also get a mouthful of drug.[38]

39. Damyanov C, et al.Low-dose chemotherapy with insulin (insulin potentiation therapy) in combination with hormone therapy for treatment of castration-resistant prostate cancer.SRN Urol. 2012;2012:140182.
40. Nixon, D. Alternative and Complementary Therapies in Oncology Care. Journal of Clinical Oncology, Vol 17, No 11S, 1999: 35-37.
41. Lipinski B, Egyud LG. Resistance of cancer cells to immune recognition and killing. Med Hypotheses. 2000 Mar;54(3):456-60.
42. Beuth J. Proteolytic enzyme therapy in evidence-based complementary oncology: fact or fiction? Integr Cancer Ther. 2008 Dec;7(4):311-6.
43. Raffaghello L, et al. Fasting and differential chemotherapy protection in patients. Cell Cycle. 2010 Nov 15; 9(22): 4474–4476.
44. Poff AM, Ari C, et al. Ketone supplementation decreases tumor cell viability and prolongs survival of mice with metastatic cancer. Int J Cancer. 2014 Oct 1; 135(7): 1711–1720.
45. Cellarier E, et al. Methionine dependency and cancer treatment. Cancer Treat Rev. 2003 Dec;29(6):489-99.
46. "NORI" is an acronym for the Nutritional Oncology Research Institute, where this protocol was developed. A central feature of this diet is restriction of the amino acid, methionine, because it is needed for cancer cells to multiply.

# Chapter 15

1. Corsino L, Dhatariya K, Umpierrez G. Management of Diabetes and Hyperglycemia in Hospitalized Patients. South Dartmouth (MA): MDText.com, Inc.; 2000-2014 Oct 4.
2. Levinthal, G., Tavill, A. Liver Disease and Diabetes Mellitus. Clinical Diabetes. Vol. 17 #2 1999.
3. The fasting blood sugar is a measure of the glucose in the blood in the morning before having eaten anything. The hemoglobin A1C is an indirect indicator of the average blood sugar in the preceding few months.
4. In recent years, another two types of diabetes have been recognized. Type 1.5 diabetes is also known as latent autoimmune diabetes of adults (LADA), which some authors regard as a variation of type 1 diabetes that develops slowly and finally shows up when the person reaches adulthood. Type 3 diabetes involves impairment of the brain cells' ability to absorb glucose. Current thinking regards type 3 diabetes as a major driver, if not the primary driver of Alzheimer's disease.[5]
5. De la Monte SM, Wands JR. Azheimer's Disease Is Type 3 Diabetes–Evidence Reviewed. J Diabetes Sci Technol. 2008 Nov; 2(6): 1101–1113.

6. Birgisdottir BE, et. al. Lower consumption of cow milk protein A1 beta-casein at 2 years of age, rather than consumption among 11- to 14-year-old adolescents, may explain the lower incidence of type 1 diabetes in Iceland than in Scandinavia. Ann Nutr Metab. 2006;50(3):177-83.

7. Schliess F, von Dahl S, Haussinger D. Insulin Resistance Induced by Loop Diuretics and Hyperosmolarity in Perfused Rat Liver. Biol Chem. 2001 July; 382(7):1063-9.

8. Smith GI, et al. Muscle Insulin Resistance Independent of Leucine-Mediated mTOR Activation. Diabetes. 2015 May;64(5):1555-63. doi: 10.2337/db14-1279. Epub 2014 Dec 4.

9. Newgard, C.B. An, J. Baine, J.R., et al. A branched chain-amino acid metabolic signature that differentiates obese and lean humans and contributes to insulin resistance. Cell Metabolism. 2009; 9(4): 311-26.

10. Viguiliouk, E. et al. Effect of Replacing Animal Protein with Plant Protein on Glycemic Control in Diabetes: A Systematic Review and Meta-Analysis of Randomized Controlled Trials. Nutrients. 2015 Dec; 7(12): 9804–9824.

11. Allen, N.E. et al. Life-style determinants of serum insulin-like growth factor-1 (IGF-1), C-peptide and hormone binding protein levels in British Women. Cancer Causes and Control. .2003; 14(1): 65-74.

12. Hancock CR, Han DH, Chen M, Terada S, Yasuda T, Wright DC, Holloszy JO. High-fat diets cause insulin resistance despite an increase in muscle mitochondria. Proc Natl Acad Sci U S A. 2008 Jun 3;105(22):7815-20.

13. Lovejoy J. C. The influence of dietary fat on insulin resistance. Curr Diab Rep. 2002 Oct;2(5):435-40.

14. Corcoran, M.P. Lamon-Fava, S. Fielding, R.A. Skeletal muscle lipid deposition and insulin resistance: effect of dietary fatty acids and exercise. Am J Clin Nutr March 2007 85: 662-677.

15. Barnard N.D. Dr. Neal Barnard's Program for reversing diabetes. Rodale Books, NY New York. 39-57.

16. Sweeney J. Dietary Factors that Influence the dextrose tolerance test: A preliminary Study. 1927; 40818.

17. Holt H, Miller JC, Petocz P. Insulin Index of Foods: the insulin demand generated by 100kj portions of common foods. Am J Cli Nutri. 1997. 66:1264-1267.

18. Kiehm TG, Anderson JW, Ward K. Beneficial effects of a high carbohydrate, high fiber diet on hyperglycemic diabetic men. American Journal of Clinical Nutrition. August 1976 29: 895.

19. Anderson JW, Ward K. High-carbohydrate, high-fiber diets for insulin-treated men with diabetes mellitus Am J Clin Nutr November 1979 32: 2312-2321.

20. Hancock CR, Han DH, Chen M, Terada S, Yasuda T, Wright DC, Holloszy JO. High-fat diets cause insulin resistance despite an

increase in muscle mitochondria. Proc Natl Acad Sci U S A. 2008 Jun 3;105(22):7815-20.

21. Kuršvietienė L., et al. Multiplicity of effects and health benefits of resveratrol. Medicina (Kaunas). 2016;52(3):148-55.

22. Meyer, B, J, et al. Some Biochemical Effects of a Mainly Fruit Diet in Man. Department of Physiology, University of Pretoria and Atomic Energy Board, and A. C. Meyer, Medical Research Council Pretoria. March 6, 1071.

23. Jenkin, D.A., et al. Effect of a very-high-fiber vegetable, fruit, and nut diet on serum lipids and colonic function. Metabolism (Impact Factor: 3.89). 04/2001; 50(4):494-503. DOI: 10.1053/meta.2001.21037. St. Michael's Hospital, Toronto, Quebec, Canada.

24. (No specific author listed). Written by the staff of the Center for Human Nutrition and the Department of Internal Medicine and Clinical Nutrition, University of Texas Southwestern Medical Center, and Department of Veterans Affairs Medical Center, Dallas 75235-9052, USA. High-monounsaturated-fat diets for patients with diabetes mellitus: a meta-analysis. Am J Clin Nutr. 1998 Mar;67(3 Suppl):577S-582S.

25. Barnard, N.D., et al. A low-fat vegan diet and a conventional diabetes diet in the treatment of type 2 diabetes: a randomized, controlled, 74-wk clinical trial. Am J Clin Nutr. 2009 May; 89(5): 1588S–1596S.

26. Villegas, R., et al. Legume and soy food intake and the incidence of type 2 diabetes in the Shanghai Women's Health Study. Am J Clin Nutr. 2008 Jan; 87(1): 162–167.

27. Tricia Y., et al. Regular Consumption of Nuts Is Associated with a Lower Risk of Cardiovascular Disease in Women with Type 2 Diabetes1,2. Nutr. 2009 Jul; 139(7): 1333–1338.

28. Asif, M. The prevention and control the type-2 diabetes by changing lifestyle and dietary pattern. J Educ Health Promot. 2014; 3: 1. Published online 2014 Feb 21.

29. Private correspondence with Howard Silverman Ph.D. D.C.

30. Blesso CN, Et al. Whole egg consumption improves lipoprotein profiles and insulin sensitivity to a greater extent than yolk-free egg substitute in individuals with metabolic syndrome. metabol.2012.08.014.

31. Tanasescu M1, et al. Dietary fat and cholesterol and the risk of cardiovascular disease among women with type 2 diabetes. Am J Clin Nutr. 2004 Jun;79(6):999-1005.

32. Bazzano LA, Li TY, et al. Intake of Fruit, Vegetables, & Fruit Juices & Risk of Diabetes in Women. Diabetes Care 2008;31:1311-1317.

33. Carter P, Gray LJ, Troughton J, et al. Fruit and vegetable intake and incidence of type 2 diabetes mellitus: systematic review and meta-analysis. BMJ 2010;341:c4229.

34. Li S, et al. Fruit intake decreases risk of incident type 2 diabetes: an updated meta-analysis. Endocrine. 2015 Mar;48(2):454-60. doi: 10.1007/s12020-014-0351-6. Epub 2014 Jul 30.
35. Risérus, U., et al. Dietary fats, and prevention of type 2 diabetes. Prog Lipid Res. 2009 Jan; 48(1): 44–51.
36. Lee, C.T, et al. Egg consumption and insulin metabolism in the Insulin Resistance Atherosclerosis Study. Public Health Nutr. 2014 Jul;17(7):1595-602.
37. Barnard, N., et al. Meat Consumption as a Risk Factor for Type 2 Diabetes. Nutrients. 2014 Feb; 6(2): 897–910.

## Chapter 16

1. Parker JC, et al. Pathobiologic features of human candidiasis. A common deep mycosis of the brain, heart and kidney in altered host. Am j of clin pathology. 65(6), 991-1000.
2. White S, Larsen B. Candida albicans morphogenesis is influenced by estrogen. Cellular and Molecular Life Sciences CMLS. October 1997, Volume 53, Issue 9, pp 744–749.
3. Plotner B. Five factors that Perpetuate Candida. Dec, 12 2013. From website: Nourishingplot.com.
4. From Body Ecology website: Bodyecology.com

## Chapter 18

1. Bazzan A, et al. Multi-nutrient supplement improves hormone ratio associated with cancer risk. J Transl Med. 2013; 11: 252.
2. Godfrey RJ, et al. The exercise-induced growth hormone response in athletes. Sports Med. 2003;33(8):599-613.
3. Chen P., et al. Lycopene and Risk of Prostate Cancer: A Systematic Review and Meta-Analysis. Medicine (Baltimore). 2015 Aug;94(33).
4. Preuss HG, et al. Randomized trial of a combination of natural products (cernitin, saw palmetto, B-sitosterol, vitamin E) on symptoms of benign prostatic hyperplasia (BPH). Int Urol Nephrol. 2001;33(2):217-25.

## Chapter 19

1. Brain cells can also generate some of their energy from burning ketone bodies, which are essentially chunks of unburned fat molecules. Ketone bodies are produced when other body cells burn fats so rapidly that they cannot absorb oxygen fast enough to completely break down fat molecules into carbon dioxide and water.
2. Tomljenovic L. Aluminum and Alzheimer's disease: is there a plausible link? J Alzheimers Dis. 2011;23: 567-98.
3. Aluminum is used as an adjuvant in some vaccines.
4. Luke J. Fluoride deposition in the aged human pineal gland. Caries Res. 2001 Mar-Apr;35(2):125-8.

5. (No author) Association of lifetime exposure to fluoride and cognitive functions in Chinese children: A pilot study. Neurotoxicology and Teratology. January-February 2015.

6. Beilharz, J., et al. Diet-Induced Cognitive Deficits: The Role of Fat and Sugar, Potential Mechanisms and Nutritional Interventions. Nutrients. 2015 Aug; 7(8): 6719–6738.

7. Mailman T, Hariharan M, Karten B. Inhibition of neuronal cholesterol biosynthesis with lovastatin leads to impaired synaptic vesicle release even in the presence of lipoproteins or geranylgeraniol. *J Neurochem.* 2011;119(5):1002-1015.

8. Olié E, Picot MC, Guillaume S, Abbar M, Courtet P. Measurement of total serum cholesterol in the evaluation of suicidal risk. J Affect Disord. 2011 Apr 25.

9. Haag M. Essential fatty acids and the brain Can J Psychiatry 2003;48(3):195-203.

10. Mortensen EL; Michaelsen KF; Sanders SA; Reinisch JM. The association between duration of breast-feeding and adult intelligence. JAMA 2002;287(18):2365-2371.

11. Helland IB, et al. Maternal supplementation with very-long-chain n-3 fatty acids during pregnancy and lactation augments children's IQ at 4 years of age. Pediatrics 2003;111(1):e39-40.

12. Tuppo EE, Forman LJ. Free radical oxidative damage and Alzheimer's disease. J Am Osteopath Assoc. 2001 Dec;101.

13. Smith, MA, et al. Increased Iron and Free Radical Generation in Preclinical Alzheimer Disease and Mild Cognitive Impairment. J of Alzheimers's Disease, vol 19, no. 1 pp 363-372, 21010.

14. Giem P, et al. The incidence of dementia and intake of animal products: preliminary findings from the Adventist Health Study. Neuroepidemiology. 1993;12(1):28-36.

15. Bested AC. et al. Intestinal microbiota, probiotics, and mental health: from Metchnikoff to modern advances: Part II – contemporary contextual research. Gut Pathology. 2013. 5:3.

16. Ifflu-Soltesz Z. el at. Influence of prolonged fasting on monoamineoxidase and semicarbazide-sensitive amino oxidase activity in rats white adipose tissue. J of Physiological Biochemistry. 2099 March;65(1):1123.

17. Jäger A.K., Saaby L. Flavonoids and the CNS. Molecules 2011, 16.

18. Yoshino S, et al. Effect of quercetin and glucuronide metabolites on the monoamine oxidase-A reaction in mouse brain mitochondria. Nutrition. 2011. Jul-Aug;27(7-8):847-52.

19. Binh Nguyen, et al. Fruit and vegetable consumption and psychological distress: cross-sectional and longitudinal analyses based on a large Australian sample. BMJ Open. 2017; 7(3): e014201.

20. Orlich MJ, et al. Vegetarian Dietary Patterns and Mortality in Adventist Health Study. JAMA Intern Med. 2013 Jul 8; 173(13): 1230–1238.
21. Poulose SM, et al. Role of walnuts in maintaining brain health with age. J Nutr. 2014 Apr;144(4 Suppl):561S-566S.
22. Valverde M E. et al. Edible Mushrooms: Improving Human Health and Promoting Quality Life. Int J Microbiol. 2015; 2015: 376387. Int J Med Mushrooms. 2013;15(6):539-54.
23. Lai PL, et al. Neurotrophic properties of the Lion's mane medicinal mushroom, Hericium erinaceus (Higher Basidiomycetes) from Malaysia. Int J Med Mushrooms. 2013;15(6):539-54.

# Chapter 20

1. Rao U. Links between depression and substance abuse in adolescents: neurobiological mechanisms. Am J Prev Med. 2006 Dec;3.
2. Strickland PL, Deakin JF, Percival C, Dixon J, Gater RA, Goldberg DP. Bio-social origins of depression in the community. Interactions between social adversity, cortisol, and serotonin neurotransmission. Br J Psychiatry. 2002 Feb;180:168-73.
3. Albsi. M Stress and Addiction. Biological and Physychological Mechanisms. Academic Press. 2007. P 25.
4. Khalid S, et al. Effects of Acute Blueberry Flavonoids on Mood in Children and Young Adults, Nutrients. 2017 Feb; 9(2): 158
5. Jäger A.K., Saaby L. Flavonoids and the CNS. Molecules 2011, 16, 1471-1485.
6. Colin A, Reggers J, et al. Lipids, depression and suicide. Encophale 2003; 29: 49-58.
7. Sagducu K, Dokucu ME, et al. Omega-3 fatty acids decreased irritability of patients with bipolar disorder in an add-on, open label study. Nutrition Journal (2005); 4:6.
8. Olié E, Picot MC, Guillaume S, Abbar M, Courtet P. Measurement of total serum cholesterol in the evaluation of suicidal risk. J Affect Disord. 2011 Apr 25.
9. Wolfe AR, Arroyo C, Tedders SH, Li Y, Dai Q, Zhang J. Epub 2010 Nov 23. Dietary protein and protein-rich food in relation to severely depressed mood: A 10 year follow-up of a national cohort. Neuropsychopharmacol Biol Psychiatry. 2011 Jan 15;35(1):232-8.
10. Armstrong, D.J. et al. Vitamin D Deficiency is Associated with Depression and Fibromyalgia. Clinical Rheumatology. Volume 26, Number 4, 551-554.
11. Kouchakoff P. The influence of food on the blood formula of man. 1st International Congress of Microbiology II. Paris (France): Masson & Cie; 1930. p. 490–3.

12. Pottenger F. The effect of heat-processed foods and metabolized vitamin D milk on the entofacial structures of experimental animals. Am J Orthod Oral Surg 1946;32:467–85.
13. Goeders NE. The impact of stress on addiction. Eur Neuropsychopharmacol. 2003 Dec;13(6):435-41.
14. Sinha, R. Chronic Stress, Drug and Vulnerability to Addiction. Ann NY Acad Sci. Oct 2008; 1141: 105-130.
15. Jukić T, et al. The use of a food supplementation with D-phenylalanine, L-glutamine and L-5-hydroxytriptophan in the alleviation of alcohol withdrawal symptoms. Coll Antropol. 2011 Dec;35(4):1225-30.
16. Kanarek RB. Artificial food dyes and attention deficit hyperactivity disorder. Nutr Rev. 2011 Jul;69(7):385-91.

## Chapter 21

1. Hemenway, T. Gaia's Garden, pg 71. Chelsey Green Pub Co, 2000.
2. Hemenway, T. Gaia's Garden, pg 72. Chelsey Green Pub Co, 2000.
3. Paraphrase of the famous words of Dr. Martin Luther King Jr. "An injustice anywhere is an injustice everywhere."
4. Lowenfels J and Lewis W. Teaming with Microbes.
5. Pollan M. The Omnivore's Dilemma pgs 145. Penguin Books, 2006.
6. Damalas, CA. Eleftherohorinos, IG. Pesticide Exposure, Safety Issues, and Risk Assessment Indicators. Nt J Environ Res Health. May 2011; 8(5): 1402-1419.
7. Wake, DB, Vredenburg, VY. Are we in the midst of the 6th great extinction? Proc Natl Acad Sci U S A. 2008 Aug 12; 105.
8. Fukuoka, M, et al. The One-Straw Revolution: An Introduction to Natural Farming. Chelsea Green Publising. Sept 14. 2015.
9. Lynn Jones, manager of Nacogdoches Farmer's Market.

## Appendix A

1. Khawaja O, et al. Egg Consumption and Incidence of Heart Failure: A Meta-Analysis of Prospective Cohort Studies. Front Nutr. 2017; 4: 10.
2. Hobbs GJ, et al. Association between egg consumption and cardiovascular disease events, diabetes, and all-cause mortality. Eur J Nutr. 2017 Nov 2.
3. Djuosse L and Gaziano M. Egg Consumption and Cardiovascular Disease and Mortality The Physicians' Health Study. Am J Clin Nutr. 2008 Apr; 87(4): 964–969.
4 Shin JY, et al. Egg consumption in relation to risk of cardiovascular disease and diabetes: a systematic review and meta-analysis. Am J Clin Nutr. 2013 Jul; 98(1): 146–159.
5. Blesso CN, Et al. Whole egg consumption improves lipoprotein profiles and insulin sensitivity to a greater extent than yolk-free egg

substitute in individuals with metabolic syndrome. metabol.2012.08.014.

6.Tanasescu M1, et al. Dietary fat and cholesterol and the risk of cardiovascular disease among women with type 2 diabetes. Am J Clin Nutr. 2004 Jun;79(6):999-1005.

## Appendix B

1. U.S. Public Law C. Food Allergen Labelling And Consumer Protection Act of 2004. Public Law 2004; 108-282:905-11.
2. Douglas CC, Johnson SA, Arjmandi BH. Soy and its isoflavones: the truth behind the science in breast cancer. Anticancer Agents Med Chem. 2013 Oct;13(8):1178-87.
3. Xiao-Xing Chi· and Tao Zhang. The effects of soy isoflavone on bone density in north region of climacteric Chinese women. J Clin Biochem Nutr. 2013 Sep; 53(2): 102–107.
4. Patisaul HB, and Jefferson W. The pros and cons of phytoestrogens. Neuroendocrinol. 2010 Oct; 31(4): 400–419.
5. Roccisano D, et al. A possible cause of Alzheimer's dementia - industrial soy foods. Med Hypotheses. 2014 Mar;82(3):250-4.

## Appendix C

1. Blue, L. Salt: How Bad Is It, Really? July 12, 2011.
2. Lelong H, et al. Relationship Between Nutrition and Blood Pressure: A Cross-Sectional Analysis from the NutriNet-Santé Study, a French Web-based Cohort Study. Am J of Hypertension. Volume 28, Issue 3, 1 March 2015, Pages 362–371.
3. Ellison D.H. and Terker A.S. Why Your Mother Was Right: How Potassium Intake Reduces Blood Pressure. Trans Am Clin Climatol Assoc. 2015; 126: 46–55.
4. Hyunwoo O, et al. Low Salt Diet and Insulin Resistance. Clin Nutr Res. 2016 Jan; 5(1): 1-6
5. Other studies indicate that high levels of sodium can increase insulin resistance. (see reference #8 below).
6. Private correspondence.
7. Edwards DG, Farquhar WB. Vascular Effects of Dietary Salt. Curr Opin Nephrol Hypertens. Curr Opin Nephrol Hypertens. 2015 Jan; 24(1): 8–13. .
8. Baudrand R, et al. High sodium intake is associated with increased glucocorticoid production, insulin resistance and metabolic syndrome. Clin Endocrinol (Oxf). 2014 May;80(5):677-84.

## Appendix E

1. Hancock C.R, et al. High-fat diets cause insulin resistance despite an increase in muscle mitochondria. Proc Natl Acad Sci. 2008. Jun 3;105(22): 7815–20.
2. Blaylock, Russell L. Health and Nutrition Secrets that can Save Your Life. Albuquerque, NM. Health Press, 2006. Pp 293–294

3. Vogel, R. Brachial Artery Ultrasound. A Nonvasive Tool in Assessment of Triglyceride Rich Lipoproteins. Clinical Cardiology. June 1999.
4. Intahphuak S, et al. Anti-inflammatory, analgesic, and antipyretic activities of virgin coconut oil. Pharm Biol. 2010 Feb;48(2):151-7.
5. Nevin KG, Rajamohan T. Effect of topical application of virgin coconut oil on skin components and antioxidant status during dermal wound healing in young rats. Skin Pharmacol Physiol. 2010;23(6):290-7. Faizal C, et al. Effect of coconut oil in plaque related gingivitis — A preliminary report, Niger Med J. 2015 Mar-Apr; 56(2): 143–147.

## Appendix F

1. Seow-Choen, S. The physiology of colonic hydrotherapy. Colorectal Dis. 2009 Sep;11(7):686-8.
2. (No author). Adverse effects after medical, commercial, or self-administered colon cleaning procedures. National Collaborating Centre for Environmental Health at the British Columbia Centre for Disease Control, January 2018.
3. Taffinder NJ, et al. Retrograde commercial colonic hydrotherapy. Colorectal Dis. 2004 Jul;6(4):258-60.
4. Carter GT, et al. Side effects of commonly prescribed analgesic medications. Phys Med Rehabil Clin N Am. 2014 May;25(2):457-70.
5. Polter D. Risk of colon perforation during colonoscopy at Baylor University Medical Center, Proc (Bayl Univ Med Cent). 2015 Jan; 28(1): 3–6.

## Appendix G

1. Meredith, SE. et al. A Comprehensive Review and Research Agenda. J Caffeine Res. 2013 Sep; 3(3): 114–130.
2. From the Gerson Institute website.
3. White BC, et al. Anxiety and muscle tension as consequences of caffeine withdrawal. Science. 1980 Sep 26;209(4464):1547-8.
4. Hurley CF, et al. The effect of caffeine ingestion on delayed onset muscle soreness. J Strength Cond Res. 2013 Nov;27(11):3101-9.
5. Cooper C, et al. Is caffeine consumption a risk factor for osteoporosis? Curr Diabetes Rev. 2012 May;8(3):162-8.
6. Boekema PJ, et al. Coffee and gastrointestinal function: facts and fiction. A review. Scand J Gastroenterol Suppl. 1999;230:35-9.
7. Cheryl D. Conrad. Chronic Stress-Induced Hippocampal Vulnerability: The Glucocorticoid Vulnerability Hypothesis. Rev Neurosci. 2008; 19(6): 395–411.
8. Nehlig A. Effects of coffee/caffeine on brain health and disease: What should I tell my patients? Pract Neurol. 2016 Apr;16(2):89-95. doi: 10.1136/practneurol-2015-001162.
9. Butt MS, Sultan MT. Coffee and its consumption: benefits and risks. Crit Rev Food Sci Nutr. 2011 Apr;51(4):363-73.

10. Muley A[1], et al. Coffee to reduce risk of type 2 diabetes?: a systematic review. Curr Diabetes Rev. 2012 May;8(3):162-8.

## Appendix H

1. Levine M, et al. Ascorbic acid & in situ kinetics: a new approach to vitamin requirements Am J Clin Nutr Dec 1991 54:1157S-1162S.
2. Milton, K (2003). "Micronutrient intakes of wild primates: are humans different?" Comparative Biochemistry and Physiology. 136 (1): 47–59.
3. Rath, M. Why Animals Don't Get Heart Attacks, but People Do! Dr. Rath Education Services. Page 14.
4. Forastiere F, et al. Consumption of Vitamin C in Fresh Fruit and Wheezing Symptoms in Children. SIDRIA Collective Group. Thorax 2000:55(4): 283-8

# Food as Medicine Index

This index serves as a quick reference to the pages that describe nutritional support for a given condition.

# General Index

## A

Acai Berries, 39
Acidifying and alkalizing foods, 31
Acne, 77
Addiction, 117, 182, 187, 188
Age spots, 77
Alcohol, 97, 169
Allergies, 68, 69, 71, 72, 75, 84, 86,
Almonds, 39
Aloe Vera, 39, 79, 106
Aluminum, 169
Angina pectoris, 93
Antibiotics, 118, 146
Anti-fungal Agents, 147
Antioxidants, 33, 34
Apples, 37, 123, 124, 128
Arthritis, 31, 37, 57, 86, 97, 101,
105, 106, 116, 221
Asparagus, 36, 38
Athletes foot, 77, 82
Autoimmune, 115, 116
Avocados, 68, 125

## B

B vitamins, 45, 63, 88, 91, 92, 98,
Bananas, 37, 123, 171
Beets, 38, 123
Blackberries, 35, 124, 128
Blueberries, 37, 124
Brain, 163, 167, 168, 169, 170-187
Brain-Balancing Diet, 177
Broccoli, 36, 38, 123, 124, 228
Bronchitis, 74
Building foods and cleansing
foods, 31, 56

## C

Caffeine, 88, 97, 103, 137, 168, 187,
212, 213, 223, 237
Calcium, 92, 224
Cancer, 15, 16, 28, 31, 34, 35, 56, 57,
61, 62, 84, 110, 121, 122, 123, 124,
125, 126, 127, 128, 129, 130, 131,
132, 138, 151, 156, 159.
Carbohydrates, 24, 25, 133, 137,
140, 153
Cardiovascular disease, 107
Carrots, 38, 164
Celery, 38
Cholesterol, 107, 109, 111, 113, 114,
137, 185, 201
Coconut oil, 44, 68, 79, 154, 222
Colon Cancer, 64, 221
Colonic irrigation, 210
Colostrum, 40
Common Cold, 74
Cortisone, 44, 103

## D

Dairy, 30
Dandelion greens, 38
Dehydration, 137
Depression, 37, 65, 84, 97, 117, 135,
145, 159, 170, 172, 173, 174, 175,
184, 185, 186, 188,
Dermatitis, 77, 78, 79, 80
Dermis, 78, 79, 80, 81
DHA, 173, 174, 184
Diabetes Mellitus, 122, 133, 135,
229
Digestion, 61, 62
Diverticulosis, 64
Dry fast, 52

# E

Eczema,, 77
Eggs, 30, 199, 208
Emphysema, 74
Enema, 210, 211
EPA, 174, 184
Epidermis, 78, 79
Exercise, 89, 96, 104, 106, 114, 137, 142, 157, 164, 165, 186, 224
Exfoliation, 81

# F

Fasting, 48, 49, 51, 130, 135, 176, 220, 221, 230, 234
Fats, 98, 106, 110, 118, 138, 142, 154, 155, 156, 173, 217
Fermentative bacteria, 63
Fermented Foods, 148
Fiber, 140
Fibromyalgia, 94, 95
Figs, 37
Flavonoids, 92, 114, 124, 125, 172, 183, 184
Flax seeds, 34
Flax seeds, 39, 142
Food as Medicine, 1, 33, 41, 54
Food Combining, 65, 67, 221
Food Groups, 23, 28
Foods that Heal, 37
Fruit, 28, 139, 140, 142, 157, 227

# G

Garlic, 75, 123, 125, 165
General Adaptation Syndrome, 84
Ginger, 75
Ginkgo Biloba, 113
Glutathione, 33, 36
Glycemic index, 139, 140, 217
Goji Berries, 40
Gout, 105

Grains, 28, 97, 146, 187

# H

Heart Attack, 107
Hemorrhoids, 63
Hippocrates, 11, 12, 41
Hormones, 134, 159, 160, 162, 164, 165

# I

Immune System, 115, 118, 119
Inflammation, 33, 34, 74, 93, 219, 222, 224
Inflammatory bowel disease (IBD, 64
Influenza, 74
Insulin Resistance, 136, 230, 232
Intestinal Bacteria, 62
Irritable bowel syndrome (IBS, 63

# J

James Watson & Francis Crick, 17
Jock itch, 77, 145

# K

Kale, 35, 38
keratin, 78, 79, 81
ketogenic diet, 131, 132, 177
Kiwi fruit, 37

# L

Leaky gut syndrome, 64
Legumes, 28
Lion's main mushroom,, 179
Liver, 70

## M

Macronutrients, 24
Magnesium, 92
maintenance diet, 16, 45, 46, 54, 69, 177
Massage Therapy, 90
Meat, 29
Mercury, 169
metabolism, 92, 105, 118, 155
Micronutrients, 24
Minerals, 24, 92
MSG (monosodium glutamate, 89, 97, 137, 169, 187
Multiple sclerosis, 116
Mushrooms, 179

## N

N-acetyl cysteine, 75
nail fungus, 77, 82, 145
Neurotoxins, 167, 168
Nitric oxide, 33, 35
Noni juice, 75
Noni Juice, 39
nuts and seeds, 29, 31, 56, 68, 69, 103, 112, 113, 141, 142, 179
Nuts and Seeds, 29, 39

## O

Obesity, 151
Obstacles to Clear Thinking, 14
osteoarthritis, 105
Osteoarthritis, 105, 224
Osteoporosis, 101, 102, 103, 104, 224
    causes, 103

## P

Papaya, 36, 37, 216
Parkinson's disease, 184

Peptic ulcers, 63
Phytonutrients, 70, 140, 152
Phytonutrients, 24, 172, 178
Pimples, 78
Pineapples, 37, 216
Pneumonia, 74
Pomegranates, 35, 37, 125
Portals of Elimination, 55, 56
Potassium, 92
Probiotics, 119, 147, 221
Protein, 24, 25, 97, 138, 153, 220, 223, 224, 230
Prunes, 37
Psoriasis, 37, 77, 78, 79, 80, 145
Pumpkin, 39
Putrefactive bacteria, 62

## R

Raspberries, 35, 124, 128, 129
Raynaud's syndrome, 94
Red or purple, 37
Reductionist Thinking Gone Bad, 14
Respiratory Cures, 71, 75
Respiratory problems, 71
Rheumatoid arthritis, 105

## S

Sanity and Sanitation, 167, 175
Saturated Fat, 110
Saturated fats, 138
Sea vegetation, 203
Sesame seeds, 39
Sinuses, 72, 73, 75
Skin cancer, 77, 79, 80
Sodium, 97
Soil, 17, 38, 121, 127, 191, 193, 194, 195, 196, 198
Sources of Toxicity, 57
Spinach, 35, 36, 38
St. John's wart, 92, 184

Strawberries, 37, 123
Stress, 84
Stress Begets More Stress, 83, 86
Sunburn, 78

## T

Toxins, 201
Tuberculosis, 74

## V

Vegetables, 29, 34, 35, 38, 126, 127, 145, 148, 227, 232
Vitamin, 63, 98, 104, 106, 110, 113, 114, 119, 186, 221

Vitamin B$_{12}$, 63
Vitamin C, 92, 103, 104, 114, 119, 207, 214, 219, 226
Vitamins, 24, 224

## W

Walnuts, 35, 39
Watermelon, 36, 37
Weight Loss, 151
Whole Foods, 26

## Y

Yeast, 145, 146
Yeast and Fungus, 145

# About the Author

Rudy Scarfalloto received his Bachelor of Science degree in biology at Brooklyn College, and his Doctor of Chiropractic degree at Life Chiropractic College. He also holds a diplomate in Clinical Nutrition from the College of Clinical Nutrition, and a diplomate in Clinical Nutrition from the Chiropractic Board of Clinical Nutrition. His other books are *The Dance of Opposites, The Edge of Time, Nutrition for Massage Therapists,* and *What Should I Eat? Book 1 and What Should I Eat? Book 2.*

Made in the USA
Columbia, SC
13 March 2024